T0214432

Lecture Notes in Computer Science   11074

Commenced Publication in 1973
Founding and Former Series Editors:
Gerhard Goos, Juris Hartmanis, and Jan van Leeuwen

More information about this series at http://www.springer.com/series/7412

Florian Knoll · Andreas Maier
Daniel Rueckert (Eds.)

Machine Learning for Medical Image Reconstruction

First International Workshop, MLMIR 2018
Held in Conjunction with MICCAI 2018
Granada, Spain, September 16, 2018
Proceedings

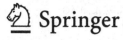 Springer

Editors
Florian Knoll [ID]
New York University
New York, NY
USA

Daniel Rueckert [ID]
Imperial College London
London
UK

Andreas Maier [ID]
University of Erlangen-Nuremberg
Erlangen
Germany

ISSN 0302-9743   ISSN 1611-3349   (electronic)
Lecture Notes in Computer Science
ISBN 978-3-030-00128-5   ISBN 978-3-030-00129-2   (eBook)
https://doi.org/10.1007/978-3-030-00129-2

Library of Congress Control Number: 2018953025

LNCS Sublibrary: SL6 – Image Processing, Computer Vision, Pattern Recognition, and Graphics

This Springer imprint is published by the registered company Springer Nature Switzerland AG
The registered company address is: Gewerbestrasse 11, 6330 Cham, Switzerland

Preface

We are proud to present the proceedings of the First Workshop on Machine Learning for Medical Image Reconstruction (MLMIR), which was held on 16th September 2018 in Granada, Spain, as part of the 21st Medical Image Computing and Computer Assisted Intervention (MICCAI) conference.

Image reconstruction is currently undergoing a paradigm shift that is driven by advances in machine learning. Whereas traditionally transform-based or optimization-based methods have dominated methods for image reconstruction, machine learning has opened up the opportunity for new data-driven approaches, which have demonstrated a number of advantages over traditional approaches. In particular, deep learning techniques have shown significant potential for image reconstruction and offer interesting new approaches. Finally, machine learning approaches also offer the possibility of application-specific image reconstruction, e.g., in motion-compensated cardiac or fetal imaging.

This is supported by the success of machine learning in other inverse problems by multiple groups worldwide, with encouraging results and increasing interest. Coincidentally, this year is the centenary of the Radon transform and the 250th anniversary of the birth of Joseph Fourier. The Fourier transform and the Radon transform provide the mathematical foundation for tomography and medical imaging. It seems appropriate and timely to consider how to invert the Radon transform and Fourier transform via machine learning, and have this workshop serve as a forum to reflect this emerging trend of image reconstruction research. In this respect, it will frame a fresh new way to recharge or redefine the reconstruction algorithms with extensive prior knowledge for superior diagnostic performance.

The aim of the workshop was to drive scientific discussion of advanced machine learning techniques for image acquisition and image reconstruction, opportunities for new applications, as well as challenges in the evaluation and validation of ML-based reconstruction approaches. We were fortunate that Jong Chul Ye (KAIST) and Michael Unser (EPFL) gave fascinating keynote lectures that summarised the state of the art in this emerging field. Finally, we received 21 submissions and were able to accept 17 papers for inclusion in the workshop. The topics of the accepted papers cover the full range of medical image reconstruction problems, and deep learning dominates the machine learning approaches that are used to tackle the reconstruction problems.

July 2018

Florian Knoll
Andreas Maier
Daniel Rueckert

Organization

Workshop Organizers

Daniel Rueckert   Imperial College London, UK
Florian Knoll   New York University, USA
Andreas Maier   University of Erlangen, Germany

Scientific Programme Committee

Bernhard Kainz   Imperial College London, UK
Bho Zhu   Havard University, USA
Bruno De Man   GE, USA
Claudia Prieto   King's College London, UK
Dong Liang   Chinese Academy of Sciences, China
Enhao Gong   Stanford University, USA
Essam Rashed   British University in Egypt, Egypt
Ge Wang   Rensselaer Polytechnic Institute, USA
Greg Zaharchuk   Stanford University, USA
Guang Yang   Royal Brompton Hospital, UK
Jo Schlemper   Imperial College London, UK
Jonas Adler   Royal Institute of Technology, Sweden
Jong Chul Ye   KAIST, South Korea
Jose Caballero   Twitter, UK
Jo Hajnal   King's College London, UK
Joseph Cheng   Stanford University, USA
Mariappan Nadar   Siemens Healthcare, USA
Matthew Rosen   Havard University, USA
Michiel Schaap   HeartFlow, USA
Morteza Mardani   Stanford University, USA
Ozan Öktem   Royal Institute of Technology, Sweden
Rebecca Fahrig   Siemens Healthcare, Germany
Simon Arridge   University College London, UK
Thomas Pock   Graz University of Technology, Austria
Tobias Wuerfl   Friedrich-Alexander-University Erlangen-Nuremberg, Germany
Tolga Cukur   Bilkent University, Turkey

Contents

Deep Learning for Magnetic Resonance Imaging

Deep Learning Super-Resolution Enables Rapid Simultaneous Morphological and Quantitative Magnetic Resonance Imaging

Akshay Chaudhari[1(✉)], Zhongnan Fang[2], Jin Hyung Lee[3], Garry Gold[1], and Brian Hargreaves[1]

[1] Department of Radiology, Stanford University, Stanford, CA, USA
{akshaysc,gold,bah}@stanford.edu,
[2] LVIS Corporation, Palo Alto, CA, USA
zhongnanf@gmail.com
[3] Department of Neurology, Stanford University, Stanford, CA, USA
ljinhy@stanford.edu

Abstract. Obtaining magnetic resonance images (MRI) with high resolution and generating quantitative image-based biomarkers for assessing tissue biochemistry is crucial in clinical and research applications. However, acquiring quantitative biomarkers requires high signal-to-noise ratio (SNR), which is at odds with high-resolution in MRI, especially in a single rapid sequence. In this paper, we demonstrate how super-resolution (SR) can be utilized to maintain adequate SNR for accurate quantification of the T_2 relaxation time biomarker, while simultaneously generating high-resolution images. We compare the efficacy of resolution enhancement using metrics such as peak SNR and structural similarity. We assess accuracy of cartilage T_2 relaxation times by comparing against a standard reference method. Our evaluation suggests that SR can successfully maintain high-resolution and generate accurate biomarkers for accelerating MRI scans and enhancing the value of clinical and research MRI.

Keywords: Super-resolution · Quantitative MRI · T_2 relaxation

1 Introduction

Magnetic resonance imaging (MRI) is an excellent non-invasive diagnostic tool to accurately assess pathologies in several anatomies. However, MRI is fundamentally constrained in optimizing for either high-resolution, high signal-to-noise ratio (SNR), or low scan durations. Enhancing one of the three outcomes necessarily degrades one or both of the others. Additionally, unlike other imaging modalities, MR images are qualitative in nature and do not directly correlate to the underlying tissue physiology. While quantitative MRI may help in assessing

© Springer Nature Switzerland AG 2018
F. Knoll et al. (Eds.): MLMIR 2018, LNCS 11074, pp. 3–11, 2018.
https://doi.org/10.1007/978-3-030-00129-2_1

tissue biochemistry and longitudinal changes, biomarker accuracy is extremely sensitive to image SNR. Consequently, it is challenging to develop a single MRI method to produce high-resolution morphological images with high quantitative biomarker accuracy in a reasonable scan time, which is tolerable for patients and which ultimately limits cost of the procedure.

1.1 Background

The double-echo in steady-state (DESS) pulse sequence can generate high-resolution images with diagnostic contrast as well as the quantitative biomarker of T_2 relaxation time, in only five-minutes of scan time [1]. The T_2 relaxation time has shown to be sensitive to collagen matrix organization and tissue hydration levels, and is useful for assessing degradation of tissues such as cartilage, menisci, tendons, and ligaments [2]. DESS intrinsically produces two images with independent contrasts. The first echo of DESS (S_1) has a T_1/T_2 weighting while the second echo of DESS (S_2) has a high T_2 weighting.

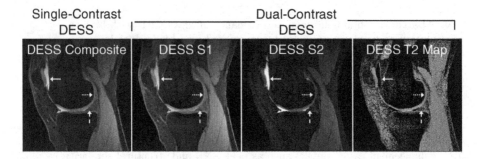

Fig. 1. Compared to the single-contrast DESS, dual-contrast DESS provides additional morphological information and automatic quantitative T_2 relaxation time maps. The separate DESS contrasts (S_1 and S_2) and T_2 maps are useful in assessing the cartilage (dashed arrow), the menisci (dotted arrow), and inflammation (solid arrow). The T_2 maps are not affected by noisy fat-suppression of bony signal.

In previous applications of DESS, the S_1 and S_2 scans are combined during the reconstruction process to produce an output with a singular contrast (herein referred as *single-contrast DESS*) [3]. However, separating the two echoes can provide considerable diagnostic utility since both echoes are sensitive to varying pathologies. Additionally, the two independent-contrast images (herein referred as *dual-contrast DESS*) can be used to analytically determine the tissue T_2 relaxation time, which is a promising biomarker for tissue degradation and OA progression [2,4]. Example images comparing the output of single-contrast DESS and dual-contrast DESS are shown in Fig. 1. Dual-contrast DESS has shown to be useful in diagnostic musculoskeletal imaging of knee as well as in research studies for evaluating OA progression [1,5].

1.2   Motivation

While promising, the dual-contrast DESS is limited in acquiring slices with 1.5 mm section-thickness to maintain adequate SNR for T_2 measurements of the cartilage and menisci. Compared to an in-plane resolution of 0.4×0.4 mm, such a high-section thickness precludes multi-planar reformations, which are essential for evaluating thin knee tissues in arbitrary planes, due to excessive image blurring. An ideal acquisition would provide sub-millimeter section thickness without biasing T_2 measurements. Advances in convolutional neural networks (CNNs) and 3D super-resolution (SR) methods may enable acquisition of slices with a thickness of 1.5 mm followed by retrospectively achieving sub-millimeter resolution, while maintaining SNR for T_2 measurements [6]. However, unlike the single-contrast DESS that has hundreds of datasets publicly available, the dual-contrast DESS is a newer sequence with very limited amounts of high-resolution data available, which makes it challenging to create a SR CNN from scratch. In such scenarios, transfer learning methods may be helpful in overcoming the limitations of a paucity of high-resolution ground-truth dual-contrast DESS training data. Specifically, it may be possible to train a SR CNN initially using single-contrast DESS datasets and subsequently adapt the network to enhance dual-contrast DESS images using limited training data.

Consequently, this study aimed to answer: **1.** Can transfer learning enhance through-plane MRI resolution for the clinically-relevant dual-contrast DESS sequence and **2.** Can transfer learning enable accurate quantitative imaging of the T_2 relaxation time by overcoming SNR limitations commonly faced in high-resolution imaging? The overall goal of this study was to evaluate whether there can be an efficient methodology to create a SR CNN for dual-contrast DESS to produce high-resolution morphological and quantitative images.

2   Related Work

Sparse-coding SR (ScSR) is a state-of-the-art non-deep-learning method that has been used for 2D MRI SR [7]. CNN-based 3D SR MRI has previously shown to transform MRI images with a high section-thickness (low slice-direction resolution) into images with lower section-thickness (high slice-direction resolution) [8]. However, this initial training was performed on single-contrast DESS sequence that does not produce quantitative biomarkers. These scans were originally acquired with a section thickness of 0.7 mm and retrospectively downsampled by a factor of 2x to a section thickness of 1.4 mm to exactly duplicate a faster, lower-resolution acquisition. The SR network was then utilized to evaluate whether the original 0.7 mm scans could be recovered from the 1.4 mm slices. We build upon these results and to extend SR to MRI sequences that can simultaneously produce multiple diagnostic contrasts and quantitative biomarkers.

3   Methods

3.1   Imaging Methodology

We utilized a CNN termed Magnetic Resonance Super-Resolution (MRSR) to extend the SR capabilities of the network initially trained for single-contrast DESS scans. The dual-contrast DESS datasets used in this study were acquired with a slice thickness of 0.7 mm (imaging parameters: $TE_1/TE_2/TR = 7/39/23$ ms, matrix size $= 416 \times 416$, field of view $= 160$ mm, flip angle $= 20°$, scan time $= 5$ min, phase encoding parallel imaging $= 2x$, slices $= 160$). A slice thicknesses of 0.7 mm was maintained for the single-contrast and dual-contrast DESS scans.

A pre-trained network for performing SR with a slice downsampling factor of 2x for the single-contrast DESS sequence was utilized to simultaneously enhance both images from the dual-contrast DESS. This pre-training was performed on image patches with input and output sizes of $32 \times 32 \times 32$ using convolutional filters of size $3 \times 3 \times 3$ and a feature map length of 64. This SR CNN network transforms an input low-resolution image into a residual image through a series of 20 convolutions and rectified linear unit (ReLU) activations [8]. An approximate high-resolution image is generated through the sum of the low-resolution input and the resultant residual using the L2-norm between the approximate and true high-resolution images as the loss function.

3.2   Transfer Learning Training for Dual-Contrast DESS

Since dual-contrast DESS contains an extra image contrast, the initial single-contrast DESS weights for the first convolution layer were duplicated to account for the dual-echoes. Similarly, the final layer output weights were modified to output two echo images instead of one, as shown in Fig. 2. In such a manner, the single-contrast DESS MRSR architecture was modified and subsequently fine-tuned to simultaneously enhance dual-contrast DESS images.

All data processing steps for the single-contrast DESS and MRSR networks were kept unchanged. This included data normalization between 0 and 1, simulation of thicker slices with a 48th-order anti-aliasing filter, a mini-batch size of 50, and a learning rate of 0.0001. All input patches had a size of $32 \times 32 \times 32 \times 2$ with a stride of 16 in the first three directions. Thus, an input image of dimensions $416 \times 416 \times 160$ was divided into 5625 patches. The MRSR network was trained for 10 epochs using 4 NVIDIA Titan 1080Ti graphical processing units.

30 dual-contrast DESS 3D datasets were used for training and 10 for validation. All datasets were collected from patients referred for a clinical MRI following institutional review board approval and informed consent, for ensuring unbiased representation of healthy and pathologic tissues.

Two unique datasets, described below, were tested using the MRSR transfer learning network because it is not currently possible to acquire a single high-resolution dataset that also has high-SNR for accurate quantitative imaging of

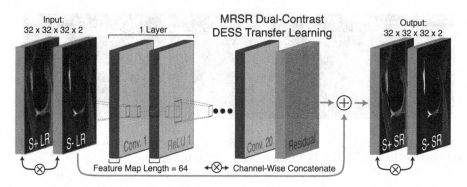

Fig. 2. The schematic of the Magnetic Resonance Super-Resolution (MRSR) network demonstrates how the low-resolution (LR) dual-contrast DESS images are simultaneously transformed into the super-resolution (SR) images.

the T_2 relaxation time. The goal of this two-fold testing was to acquire separate reference high-resolution and high-SNR scans. The dual-contrast DESS could therefore have intermediate SNR for accurate T_2 measurements and the intermediate resolution of the acquisition could be enhanced using MRSR.

Image Quality: Test Cohort 1. This dataset had identical scan parameters to the training dataset. Following the simulation of 2x thicker slices, image quality enhancements were evaluated by comparing the structural similarity (SSIM), peak SNR (pSNR), and root mean square error (RMSE) between the ground truth high-resolution and MRSR images, along with tricubic interpolated (TCI), Fourier interpolated (FI), and sparse coding super-resolution (ScSR) images.

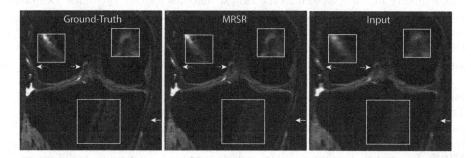

Fig. 3. MRSR coronal reformatted images demonstrate better resolution in the slice-direction (left-right) than the input TCI images, compared to the ground-truth.

T_2 Accuracy: Test Cohort 2. The second dataset had thicker slices (1.6 mm) to maintain a higher SNR for accurate T_2 quantification, since T_2 has a high sensitivity to noise [1]. Accuracy of the T_2 maps was evaluated by comparing the T_2 values in two combined adjacent slices in the medial femoral cartilage of the

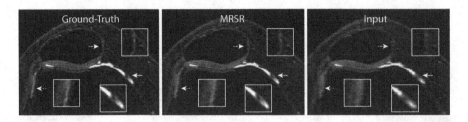

Fig. 4. Example axial reformatted MRSR images, depict finer image details considerably better than the input TCI image compared to the ground-truth.

MRSR, TCI, FI, and ScSR outputs to the ground-truth thick-slice sequences. Segmentation was performed by a reader with 5 years of experience in knee MRI segmentation. T_2 relaxation time differences, coefficients of variation (CV%), and concordance correlation coefficients (CCC) assessed T_2 variations between the methods, compared to the ground truth.

Mann-Whitney U-Tests assessed variations between morphological enhancement metrics as well as T_2 variations for all enhancement methods.

4   Results

Each epoch training duration was approximately 3 h for the total of 170,000 training patches. The SSIM, pSNR, and RMSE values between the MRSR, TCI, FI, and ScSR images to the ground-truth are shown in Table 1, where MRSR was significantly superior compared to TCI, FI, and ScSR. Comparisons for T_2 values computed with all methods are shown in Table 2. MRSR had the best image quality metrics, as well as the closest matches for the T_2 values. Despite being compared on a pixel-wise basis, which can have a high sensitivity to noise, the MRSR T_2 values had the lowest inter-method CV of 3% and an excellent CCC of 0.93. There were no statistically significant variations for T_2 for any method compared to the ground truth, likely due to a limited sample size.

Example coronal and axial images of the resolution enhancement are shown in Figs. 3 and 4. The medial collateral ligament (solid arrow, approximately 1 mm thick) is completely blurred out in the input image (Fig. 3), but can be delineated well with MRSR. Similarly, the ligament bundles (dashed arrow) and the synovium (dotted arrow) appeared blurrier in the input image than the MRSR. Figure 4 shows that signal irregularities in medial synovium (solid arrow) delineated better using MRSR than in the input image. The lateral synovial membrane (dotted arrow) also appears thickened in the blurred input image but not in the ground-truth or MRSR, which may incorrectly lead to a diagnosis of synovitis. The patellar cartilage (dashed arrow) appears blurred with diffuse signal heterogeneity in the input image, which may lead to an incorrect cartilage lesion diagnosis. Example T_2 map comparisons (shown in Fig. 5) show minimal differences between the ground-truth and MRSR images, and that the per-pixel difference map has no organized structure, suggesting minimal systematic bias.

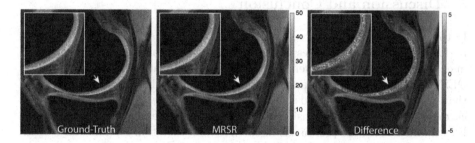

Fig. 5. MRSR T_2 relaxation time maps appear similar and provide a similar spatial distribution of T_2 values compared to the ground-truth. The difference map has no discernible structure, suggesting minimal systematic bias. (Note the different color scale). (Color figure online)

Table 1. Quantitative image quality metrics for both DESS echoes comparing the ground-truth to MRSR, TCI, FI, and ScSR images for test cohort 1. *indicates a significant difference ($p < 0.05$) compared to MRSR. †indicates that all displayed values are multiplied by 10^3.

Metric	Image	MRSR	TCI	FI	ScSR
SSIM	S_1	0.98 ± 0.01	$0.95 \pm 0.02^*$	$0.92 \pm 0.02^*$	$0.97 \pm 0.01^*$
	S_2	0.98 ± 0.01	$0.96 \pm 0.02^*$	$0.95 \pm 0.02^*$	0.97 ± 0.01
pSNR	S_1	37.7 ± 1.5	$32.5 \pm 3.6^*$	$32.4 \pm 2.8^*$	36.6 ± 1.1
	S_2	38.7 ± 2.0	33.6 ± 4.2	$33.6 \pm 3.5^*$	37.5 ± 1.6
RMSE†	S_1	0.18 ± 0.06	$0.72 \pm 0.56^*$	$0.69 \pm 0.47^*$	0.22 ± 0.05
	S_2	0.13 ± 0.04	0.51 ± 0.40	$0.47 \pm 0.34^*$	0.16 ± 0.05

Table 2. Cartilage T_2 relaxation times for MRSR, TCI, FI, and ScSR compared to the ground-truth using differences and coefficients of variation (CV%) in test cohort 2.

Subject	Ground-truth	MRSR	TCI	FI	ScSR
1	35.2	35.8	36.4	36.1	42.4
2	42.6	44.1	44.4	44.5	50.1
3	27.9	29.1	29.8	29.4	35.9
4	35.3	38.5	39.5	39.0	58.3
5	36.6	38.0	39.0	39.2	46.7
Average	35.5 ± 5.2	37.1 ± 5.4	37.8 ± 5.3	37.6 ± 5.5	46.7 ± 8.4
CV %	N/A	3.1 ± 1.8	4.5 ± 2.2	4.1 ± 2.0	18.8 ± 9.3
Difference	N/A	1.6 ± 1.0	2.3 ± 1.1	2.1 ± 1.1	11.2 ± 6.7
CCC	N/A	0.93	0.87	0.89	0.21

5   Discussion and Conclusion

In this study, we demonstrated that transfer learning can be effectively used to perform SR on MRI sequences with varied contrasts that are used clinically and in epidemiological studies, even with a small training dataset. The dual-contrast DESS sequence was able to maintain a considerably higher resolution and detail than the comparison methods. It is important to note that since the SR was carried out only in one dimension of the 3D dataset, the image enhancements in Figs. 3 and 4 are more prominent in the left-right direction anatomically, which is also the same direction of the displayed images.

The MRSR approach maintained comparable T_2 relaxation times between the ground-truth. A pixel-wise CV of 3% has shown to be adequate for use in OA studies and a CCC of over 0.90 indicated excellent reproducibility compared to the ground-truth [9]. With MRSR, slices can be acquired with a higher section thickness for accurate T_2 measurement, while enabling super-resolution for performing high-resolution MRI scans, which was not possible previously due to SNR limitations. Interestingly enough, all methods over-estimated T_2 values, likely because the thin cartilage has two major divisions (deep and superficial), where the deep cartilage has lower signal. Blurring from the superficial cartilage would increase signal in the deeper layer, leading to a higher T_2 value. Performing layer-wise T_2 values will be important in future studies.

In conclusion, we demonstrated how SR enhanced through-plane resolution in MRI and maintained quantitative accuracy of the T_2 relaxation time biomarker. MRSR outperforms conventional and state-of-the-art resolution enhancement methods and has potential for use in clinical and research studies.

References

1. Chaudhari, A.S., et al.: Five-minute knee MRI for simultaneous morphometry and T_2 relaxometry of cartilage and meniscus and for semiquantitative radiological assessment using double-echo in steady-state at 3T. J. Magn. Reson. Imaging **47**, 1328–1341 (2017)
2. Mosher, T.J., Dardzinski, B.J.: Cartilage MRI T_2 relaxation time mapping: overview and applications. Semin. Musculoskelet. Radiol. **8**, 355–368 (2004)
3. Peterfy, C.G., Schneider, E., Nevitt, M.: The osteoarthritis initiative: report on the design rationale for the magnetic resonance imaging protocol for the knee. Osteoarthritis Cartilage **16**(12), 1433–1441 (2008)
4. Sveinsson, B., Chaudhari, A., Gold, G., Hargreaves, B.: A simple analytic method for estimating T2 in the knee from DESS. Magn. Reson. Imaging **38**, 63–70 (2017)
5. Monu, U.D., Jordan, C.D., Samuelson, B.L., Hargreaves, B.A., Gold, G.E., McWalter, E.J.: Cluster analysis of quantitative MRI T_2 and $T_{1\rho}$ relaxation times of cartilage identifies differences between healthy and ACL-injured individuals at 3T. Osteoarthritis Cartilage **25**(October), 1–8 (2016)
6. Kim, J., Kwon Lee, J., Mu Lee, K.: Accurate image super-resolution using very deep convolutional networks. In: Proceedings of the IEEE Conference on Computer Vision and Pattern Recognition, pp. 1646–1654 (2016)

7. Wang, Y.H., Qiao, J., Li, J.B., Fu, P., Chu, S.C., Roddick, J.F.: Sparse representation-based MRI super-resolution reconstruction. Measurement **47**, 946–953 (2014)
8. Chaudhari, A.S., et al.: Super-resolution musculoskeletal MRI using deep learning. Magn. Reson. Med. (2018)
9. Baum, T., Joseph, G.B., Karampinos, D.C., Jungmann, P.M., Link, T.M., Bauer, J.S.: Cartilage and meniscal T2 relaxation time as non-invasive biomarker for knee osteoarthritis and cartilage repair procedures. Osteoarthritis Cartilage/OARS **21**(10), 1474–84 (2013)

ETER-net: End to End MR Image Reconstruction Using Recurrent Neural Network

Changheun Oh[1,2]([✉]) [ID], Dongchan Kim[2] [ID], Jun-Young Chung[2], Yeji Han[2], and HyunWook Park[1]

[1] Korea Advanced Institute of Science and Technology,
Daejeon 34141, Republic of Korea
choh@athena.kaist.ac.kr, hwpark@kaist.ac.kr
[2] Gachon University, Incheon 21565, Republic of Korea

Abstract. Recently, an end-to-end MR image reconstruction technique, called AUTOMAP, was introduced to simplify the complicated reconstruction process of MR image and to improve the quality of reconstructed MR images using deep learning. Despite the benefits of end-to-end architecture and superior quality of reconstructed MR images, AUTOMAP suffers from the large amount of training parameters required by multiple fully connected layers. In this work, we propose a new end-to-end MR image reconstruction technique based on the recurrent neural network (RNN) architecture, which can be more efficiently used for magnetic resonance (MR) image reconstruction than the convolutional neural network (CNN). We modified the RNN architecture of ReNet for image domain data to reconstruct an MR image from k-space data by utilizing recurrent cells. The proposed network reconstructs images from the k-space data with a reduced number of parameters compared with that of fully connected architectures. We present a quantitative evaluation of the proposed method for Cartesian trajectories using nMSE and SSIM. We also present preliminary images reconstructed from k-space data acquired in the radial trajectory.

Keywords: Image reconstruction · Neural network · End to end
RNN · AUTOMAP · ReNet

1 Introduction

In magnetic resonance imaging (MRI), k-space data is acquired using a variety of MR sequences consisting of different radiofrequency and gradient pulses. Then, by transforming the frequency information of the k-space data into spatial information, an MR image can be reconstructed. Generally, 2D or 3D Fourier transform (FT) is used for reconstruction of an MR image because the k-space is typically scanned in a Cartesian trajectory. However, relying entirely on the FT may not be sufficient for certain applications of MRI such as non-Cartesian MRI,

© Springer Nature Switzerland AG 2018
F. Knoll et al. (Eds.): MLMIR 2018, LNCS 11074, pp. 12–20, 2018.
https://doi.org/10.1007/978-3-030-00129-2_2

accelerated MRI, etc. In such cases, other iterative reconstruction techniques can be utilized to enhance the quality of MR images.

Recently, deep learning has been also applied in MRI to enhance the image quality [1–7]. Considering that MRI needs to consider multiple sources of errors due to its complex nature, including field inhomogeneity, eddy current effects, phase distortions, regridding, etc., an end-to-end reconstruction using deep learning could provide a unified solution and simplify the reconstruction process of MRI. Image reconstruction by domain-transform manifold learning (AUTOMAP) [1] was a state-of-the-art technique that performed end-to-end reconstruction. As each voxel of an MR image can be regarded as a weighted sum of the entire k-space, AUTOMAP is structured as multiple fully connected layers, requiring a large amount of weights and biases. As a result, the maximum size of input data is limited by the hardware specification that determines the amount of processable weights and biases. To resolve this issue, we adopt the bidirectional recurrent neural network (RNN) as an alternative to the fully connected layers [8,9]. As a recurrent cell has a memory that stores states, it allows the previous information to be reflected in the output of the next time step without overloading the system.

In this work, the RNN extracts features for image reconstruction while sweeping the k-space both horizontally and vertically. In addition, by utilizing the sequentiality of a recurrent cell, the bidirectional RNN can decode the input k-space data into image data with a reduced number of weights and biases than the fully connected layers. In the following sections, we present a detailed explanation of the proposed recurrent neural network architecture and experiment results.

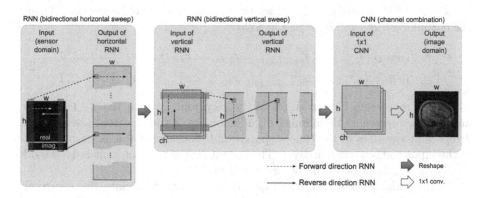

Fig. 1. The proposed network architecture. The input is sensor domain data with a dimension of $w \times h \times 2$ (2 for real and imaginary k-space). Dotted lines represent forward direction RNNs and solid lines represent reverse direction RNNs. Two RNN layers for horizontal and vertical sweeps are sequentially used to learn the relation of k-space data in the left-right, right-left, top-down, and bottom-up directions.

2   Method

2.1   Network Architectures

The proposed architecture was designed by benchmarking the ReNet architecture, which was proposed as an alternative to the use of convolutional neural network (CNN) (Fig. 1). The ReNet replaces the convolution and pooling layer of the deep CNN with four recurrent neural networks that sweep both horizontally and vertically in forward and backward directions across the images. In ReNet [9], the relationship between input patch $P = \{p_{i,j}\}$, state $z_{i,j}^F, z_{i,j}^R$, and feature map $V = \{v_{i,j}\}_{i=1,...,I}^{j=1,...,J}$, where $v_{i,j} \in \mathbb{R}^{2d}$ and d is the number of recurrent units, are defined as follows.

$$v_{i,j}^F = f_{VFWD}\left(z_{i,j-1}^F, p_{i,j}\right), for \quad j = 1, ..., J$$
$$v_{i,j}^R = f_{VREV}\left(z_{i,j+1}^R, p_{i,j}\right), for \quad j = J, ..., 1 \tag{1}$$

In this work, we modified the architecture of the original ReNet with the consideration of the characteristics of MR k-space data, thereby improve stability and convergence of network for MRI reconstruction application. In MRI, most of the high frequency values in k-space are close to zero, preventing the network from properly updating weights and biases. Similarly, the marginal areas of MR images tend to have zero-values, which is also inadequate for training. Thus, instead of using single points as an input, single columns (or rows) are used as an input to the recurrent layer. For input format of the network, complex values of the k-space data having a matrix size of $w \times h$ ($X \in \mathbb{C}^{w \times h}$) can be processed as two sets of real-value data, which can be denoted as $X = \{x_{i,j,k}\}$ for $X \in \mathbb{R}^{w \times h \times 2}$, where w is size of width (k_x) and h is size of height (k_y). Then, the output vectors can be defined as follows,

$$o_{.,j}^F = f_{VFWD}\left(s_{1,j-1}^F, ..., s_{n_{hidden},j-1}^F, x_{1,j,.}, ..., x_{I,j,.}\right), for \quad j = 1, ..., J$$
$$o_{.,j}^R = f_{VREV}\left(s_{1,j+1}^R, ..., s_{n_{hidden},j+1}^R, x_{1,j,.}, ..., x_{I,j,.}\right), for \quad j = J, ..., 1 \tag{2}$$

where $s_{.,j}$ represents hidden states of the recurrent layer in the j_{th} time step and n_{hidden} represents the number of hidden units in the recurrent layer. J and I represent the sizes of the time step axis and its orthogonal axis, respectively, of the input to the recurrent layer. The output size of the recurrent layer should be $2 \times n_{hidden}$ because of the bi-directionality.

In the proposed network, the input data initially flows into the recurrent layer which has a time step axis along the horizontal bi-directions. The output of the horizontal recurrent layer $O_{horizontal} \in \mathbb{R}^{w \times 2 \times n_{hidden}}$ is serialized into the same size as the input and depth dimensions. Then, the serialized output of the recurrent layer with horizontal time step axis flows into the second recurrent layer, which has a time step axis along the vertical bi-directions. The output of the recurrent layer with vertical time step axis $O_{vertical} \in \mathbb{R}^{h \times 2 \times n_{hidden}}$ is also serialized into the same size as the input and depth dimensions. Finally, the convolutional layer combines the data along the depth dimensions into a single data to generate a reconstructed image. We deploy a mean-squared-error between the regressed image and the ground truth image as a loss function of the proposed network and choose an optimizer RMSProp [10] with a learning rate of 0.002, momentum of 0.0, and decay of 0.9. Additionally, the learning rate annealing with a step decay is also applied. If a difference of loss values between the current epoch and the one before three epochs is smaller than the pre-determined threshold value, the learning rate is reduced to a predefined ratio.

2.2 Training Environment

Hardware. The proposed architecture was implemented using Tensorflow [11] based Keras [12] and processed by Intel(R) Core(TM) i5-8400 2.80 GHz CPU and NVIDIA Geforce GTX 1080-Ti GPU. Training the weights and biases takes approximately one hour per each epoch for 50,000 samples.

Dataset. 50,000 image samples of ILSVRC2012 [13] and ten MPRAGE images (3D-array samples) of HCP [14] datasets were used for training, validating, and testing. In addition to MR dataset (i.e., HCP images), we also included images of ILSVRC2012 as pre-training dataset to train the network architecture with input images having more diverse image characteristics. The T1-weighted MPRAGE images in HCP dataset were acquired with following parameters. $TR = 2,530$ ms, $TE = 1.15$ ms, $TI = 1,100$ ms, $FA = 7.0°$ and $BW = 651$ Hz/Px on a Siemens Skyra 3T MRI Scanner (Siemens Medical Solutions, Erlangen, Germany).

The preprocessing of dataset was conducted as follows. To convert natural images of ILSVRC2012 into grey scale images, we computed the luminance (Y) component from the RGB values of each pixel ($Y = 0.2125$ R $+ 0.7154$ G $+ 0.0721$ B) [15] using scikit-image, which is a well-known python package for image processing [16]. After the conversion, the intensity values were normalized into a range of 0 to 1. To guarantee consistency, the intensity of HCP brain images was also normalized into a range of 0 to 1. Then, data in the image domain was synthesized into k-space data using Cartesian or radial trajectories. To synthesize radial k-space data, the numbers of radial views (n_v) and readout samples (n_p) were 128 and 128, respectively. To synthesize radial k-space data, we used Berkeley Advanced Reconstruction Toolbox (BART) in MATLAB [17]. All images were resized as 128×128 to synthesize the k-space data $X \in \mathbb{C}^{w \times h}$ with $w = 128$ and $h = 128$ in Cartesian or the k-space data $X \in \mathbb{C}^{n_v \times n_p}$ with $n_v = 128$ and $n_p = 128$ in radial.

In addition, low pass filtered (LPF) k-space dataset was generated from the HCP MR images and used as an input of the proposed network, which was not included in the training dataset, to show the characteristics of the network and to compare it with 2D fast FT (FFT). LPF k-space data was generated by masking the high frequency of original k-space using the rectangular mask with a size of $w/2 \times h/2$.

2.3   Quantitative Evaluation

For quantitative evaluation, we deploy the normalized mean square error and structural similarity index [18] defined as follows.

$$nMSE = \frac{\sum_i^I \sum_i^I \left[x_{i,j}^{GT} - x_{i,j}^{PRED} \right]^2}{\sum_i^I \sum_i^I \left[x_{i,j}^{GT} \right]^2}, \tag{3}$$

$$SSIM = \frac{(2\mu_x\mu_y + C_1)(2\sigma_{xy} + C_2)}{(\mu_x^2 + \mu_y^2 + C_1)(\sigma_x^2 + \sigma_y^2 + C_2)}, \tag{4}$$

where $x_{i,j}^{GT}$ is the ground truth image and $x_{i,j}^{PRED}$ is the predicted image. Small constants C_1 and C_2 are included to avoid instability when the denominator is very close to zero.

3   Results

In Fig. 2, selected images from the entire dataset are presented for comparison, where the left column shows the ground truth images and the middle column shows the predicted results of the corresponding images using the proposed network. The difference map between the ground truth and the predicted image is also presented in the right column with amplified intensity (×5) for viewing purposes.

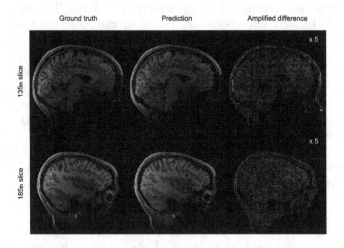

Fig. 2. Comparison of ground truth, prediction, and difference images. Upper and lower rows show the 135th and 185th slices of selected MR data of HCP, respectively. **Left** Ground truth images **Middle** Prediction images **Right** Difference between ground truth and predicted image. Magnitude of difference image is amplified with a factor of five.

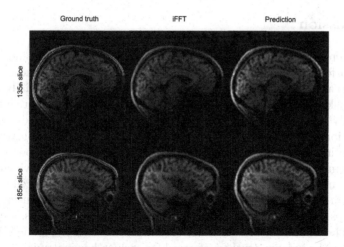

Fig. 3. Reconstruction of LPF dataset. Upper and lower rows shows the 135th and the 185th slices, respectively. **Left** Ground truth images **Middle** Inverse FFT images of LPF dataset **Right** Prediction results of LPF dataset.

As the proposed network is trained to conduct inverse FFT, we performed image reconstruction from the LPF k-space data to indirectly show the characteristics of the proposed network. Figure 3 shows the ground truth images (left column), images reconstructed using the inverse FFT (middle column), and the images reconstructed by the proposed network (right column) from the LPF k-space data. Although LPF data was not included in the training dataset, the predicted images showed blurring, which is similarly shown in the images reconstructed by inverse FFT. Thus, we speculate that the proposed network conducted similar tasks as the inverse FFT.

The mean and standard deviation of the quantitative evaluation values calculated from the entire slices of a single subject are nMSE $= 0.3399$ and SSIM $= 0.9583$. The selected 135th slice image presented in the previous figure shows nMSE of 0.4053 and SSIM of 0.9543, meaning that the selected slice represents below-average quality than the rest of the data used in this experiment. For the 185th slice, nMSE of 0.2238 and SSIM of 0.9758 were measured, representing above-average image quality.

To verify the feasibility of the proposed network for non-Cartesian trajectories, we trained and tested our network with synthesized radial data. As shown in Fig. 4, the images reconstructed by the proposed method are blurred and the edges of WM and GM are ambiguous. However, this result suggest that the proposed method may be used to end-to-end reconstruction of non-Cartesian k-space with improvements. Thus, further investigation on training process and optimization of network should be conducted to increase the quality of reconstructed images and to reduce blurring artifacts.

4   Discussion

In many deep learning techniques for image processing and understanding, CNN is preferred for the weight sharing characteristics of convolution kernel, not to mention the availability of highly optimized CNN structures. Especially in image to image tasks, the convolution kernel with locally bounded receptive field can be efficiently used. However, CNN may not be appropriate for end-to-end MR reconstruction tasks because k-space signals are integrated sum of MR signals from the entire excitation volume in MRI. For this reason, we proposed an end-to-end MR image reconstruction method based on the ReNet [9], which utilized recurrent neural network. In the proposed network, the recurrent cell has a role of collecting and holding the forward and reverse scan information using bidirectional sweeps. By utilizing information from both directional sweeps, it combines the current input and the hidden states to produce the output. As the 2D Fourier transform can be independently performed for each orthogonal axis, we designed our architecture to perform the reconstruction by sequentially using two RNNs. In the original architecture of ReNet, the recurrent cell takes input from the corresponding point or patch. However, point-by-point input data in k-space may disturb the network learning process because the magnitude of k-space data is highly unbalanced and the information is clustered in the central k-space. Thus, we modified the original architecture of ReNet, so that the recurrent cell can take input from the entire vector of the orthogonal axis to time step axis.

With respect to computation loads, the number of parameters for weights and biases in the proposed architecture is much less compared to AUTOMAP. In the custom-built version of AUTOMAP [1] architecture with an input dimension of $X \in \mathbb{R}^{2 \times n^2}$ for $n = 80$ the total number of parameters was 163,982,336. If the input dimension is increased from 80 to 128 (as in the paper), the number of parameters between the input and the first fully connected layer can be calculated as 536,887,296. Considering that this is only for the first layer of the whole architecture, it is a demanding requirement. On the other hand, the proposed network requires 79,725,073 parameters for 128×128 Cartesian k-space input of $X \in \mathbb{C}^{128 \times 128}$ and 79,733,777 parameters for 128×128 radial input of $X \in \mathbb{C}^{128 \times 128}$.

As shown in Figs. 2 and 3, predicted images show the horizontal and vertical stripe pattern artifacts, and dark regions in frontal regions. We speculate that the stripe pattern artifacts were caused by the recurrent cell used in our network architecture, and dark regions were caused by insufficient amount of training data and lack of augmentation. Thus, increasing the amount of data, improvement of augmentation algorithm, and use of more advanced activation functions, such as leaky ReLU [19] may reduce these artifacts.

In conclusion, we proposed a new end-to-end MR image reconstruction technique based on recurrent deep learning architecture. As ReNet can be used with a reduced number of training parameters, it can be used for reconstruction of images with higher resolution. In this study, preliminary results were presented to show the feasibility of ReNet for end-to-end MR image reconstruction tasks.

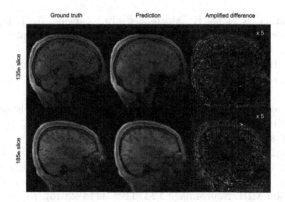

Fig. 4. Reconstructed images from radial sampling. Upper and lower rows show the 135th and the 185th slices, respectively. **Left** Ground truth images **Middle** Prediction results of radial dataset **Right** Difference between ground truth and predicted image. Magnitude of difference image is amplified with a factor of five.

Thus, further investigation should be conducted to improve image quality and to extend the proposed method for under-sampled k-space data and for other non-Cartesian trajectories.

Acknowledgment. This work was partly supported by the Brain Research Program through the National Research Foundation of Korea (NRF) funded by the Ministry of Science and ICT (NRF-2017M3C7A1047228).

References

1. Zhu, B., Liu, J.Z., Cauley, S.F., Rosen, B.R., Rosen, M.S.: Image reconstruction by domain-transform manifold learning. Nature **555**(7697), 487 (2018)
2. Han, Y., Ye, J.C.: k-space deep learning for accelerated MRI. arXiv preprint arXiv:1805.03779 (2018)
3. Hammernik, K., et al.: Learning a variational network for reconstruction of accelerated MRI data. Magn. Reson. Med. **79**(6), 3055–3071 (2018)
4. Kwon, K., Kim, D., Park, H.: A parallel MR imaging method using multilayer perceptron. Med. Phys. **44**(12), 6209–6224 (2017)
5. Schlemper, J., Caballero, J., Hajnal, J.V., Price, A.N., Rueckert, D.: A deep cascade of convolutional neural networks for dynamic MR image reconstruction. IEEE Trans. Med. Imaging **37**(2), 491–503 (2018)
6. Yang, G., et al.: DAGAN: deep de-aliasing generative adversarial networks for fast compressed sensing MRI reconstruction. IEEE Trans. Med. Imaging **37**(6), 1310–1321 (2018)
7. Quan, T.M., Nguyen-Duc, T., Jeong, W.K.: Compressed sensing MRI reconstruction using a generative adversarial network with a cyclic loss. IEEE Trans. Med. Imaging **37**(6), 1488–1497 (2018)
8. Graves, A., Schmidhuber, J.: Offline handwriting recognition with multidimensional recurrent neural networks. In: Advances in Neural Information Processing Systems, pp. 545–552 (2009)

 9. Visin, F., Kastner, K., Cho, K., Matteucci, M., Courville, A., Bengio, Y.: ReNet: a recurrent neural network based alternative to convolutional networks. arXiv preprint arXiv:1505.00393 (2015)
10. Tieleman, T., Hinton, G.: Lecture 6.5-RmsProp: divide the gradient by a running average of its recent magnitude. COURSERA: Neural Netw. Mach. Learn. **4**(2), 26–31 (2012)
11. Abadi, M., et al.: TensorFlow: a system for large-scale machine learning. OSDI **16**, 265–283 (2016)
12. Chollet, F., et al.: Keras (2015)
13. Deng, J., Berg, A., Satheesh, S., Su, H., Khosla, A., Fei-Fei, L.: ImageNet large scale visual recognition competition 2012 (ILSVRC 2012). Google Scholar (2012)
14. Fan, Q., et al.: MGH-USC human connectome project datasets with ultra-high b-value diffusion MRI. NeuroImage **124**, 1108–1114 (2016)
15. Poynton, C.: Frequently asked questions about color (1997). Accessed 19 June 2004
16. Van der Walt, S., et al.: scikit-image: image processing in python. PeerJ **2**, e453 (2014)
17. Uecker, M., et al.: Berkeley advanced reconstruction toolbox. In: Proceedings of International Society for Magnetic Resonance in Medicine, vol. 23, p. 2486 (2015)
18. Wang, Z., Bovik, A.C., Sheikh, H.R., Simoncelli, E.P.: Image quality assessment: from error visibility to structural similarity. IEEE Trans. Image Process. **13**(4), 600–612 (2004)
19. Xu, B., Wang, N., Chen, T., Li, M.: Empirical evaluation of rectified activations in convolutional network. arXiv preprint arXiv:1505.00853 (2015)

Cardiac MR Motion Artefact Correction from K-space Using Deep Learning-Based Reconstruction

Ilkay Oksuz[1]([✉]), James Clough[1], Aurelien Bustin[1], Gastao Cruz[1],
Claudia Prieto[1], Rene Botnar[1], Daniel Rueckert[2], Julia A. Schnabel[1],
and Andrew P. King[1]

[1] School of Biomedical Engineering and Imaging Sciences,
King's College London, London, UK
ilkay.oksuz@kcl.ac.uk
[2] Biomedical Image Analysis Group, Imperial College London, London, UK

Abstract. Incorrect ECG gating of cardiac magnetic resonance (CMR) acquisitions can lead to artefacts, which hampers the accuracy of diagnostic imaging. Therefore, there is a need for robust reconstruction methods to ensure high image quality. In this paper, we propose a method to automatically correct motion-related artefacts in CMR acquisitions during reconstruction from k-space data. Our method is based on the Automap reconstruction method, which directly reconstructs high quality MR images from k-space using deep learning. Our main methodological contribution is the addition of an adversarial element to this architecture, in which the quality of image reconstruction (the generator) is increased by using a discriminator. We train the reconstruction network to automatically correct for motion-related artefacts using synthetically corrupted CMR k-space data and uncorrupted reconstructed images. Using 25000 images from the UK Biobank dataset we achieve good image quality in the presence of synthetic motion artefacts, but some structural information was lost. We quantitatively compare our method to a standard inverse Fourier reconstruction. In addition, we qualitatively evaluate the proposed technique using k-space data containing real motion artefacts.

Keywords: Cardiac MR · Image reconstruction · Deep learning
UK Biobank · Image artefacts · Image quality · Automap

1 Introduction

Image reconstruction is an inverse mathematical problem for mapping the sensor domain information to the image domain. A good image reconstruction is a key component for establishing high quality images from sensors. Traditionally in MR imaging the k-space information is used in a compressed sensing framework to address the problem of image reconstruction [9]. Recently, there has been

© Springer Nature Switzerland AG 2018
F. Knoll et al. (Eds.): MLMIR 2018, LNCS 11074, pp. 21–29, 2018.
https://doi.org/10.1007/978-3-030-00129-2_3

interest in finding the mapping from the frequency domain to the image domain using deep learning techniques [10]. The majority of such methods have the aim of accelerating the image acquisition without compromising image quality. In this work, we address a different problem. We aim to correct motion artefacts with an end-to-end setup using motion artefact corrupted k-space data as the input and producing high quality images as the output.

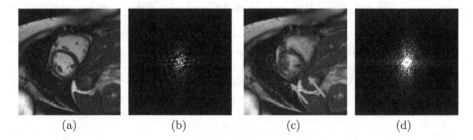

(a)   (b)   (c)   (d)

Fig. 1. Examples of a good quality CINE CMR image (a), corresponding k-space (b) and a corrupted image (c), where red arrows indicate the artefacts and the corresponding k-space (d). The k-space corruption process is able to simulate realistic motion-related artefacts. (Color figure online)

High diagnostic accuracy of image analysis pipelines requires high quality medical images. Misleading conclusions can be drawn when the original data are of low quality, in particular for cardiac magnetic resonance (CMR) imaging. CMR images can contain a range of image artefacts [2], and improving the quality of images acquired by MR scanners is a challenging problem. Traditionally, low quality images are excluded from further analysis. However, excluding images not only diminishes the research value of the cohort but also raises the issue of how to robustly and efficiently identify images for exclusion.

The UK Biobank is a large-scale study with all data accessible to researchers worldwide, and will eventually consist of CMR images from 100,000 subjects [12]. To maximize the research value of this and other similar datasets, automatic artefact correction tools are essential. One specific challenge in CMR is motion-related artefacts such as mis-triggering, arrhythmia and breathing artefacts due to incomplete breath-holds. These can result in temporal and/or spatial blurring of the images, which makes subsequent processing difficult [2]. Examples of a good quality image and a synthetic motion artefact corrupted image are shown in Fig. 1a and c for a short-axis view CINE CMR scan. The corresponding k-space data are shown in Fig. 1b and d. In this work, our goal is to recover the good quality image (Fig. 1a) from the corrupted k-space data (Fig. 1d) directly using deep learning.

Our approach is based on automatically correcting for artefacts during the reconstruction process. We use a deep neural network for correcting artefacts and evaluate our method on a synthetic dataset of 2000 2D+time CMR images from the UK Biobank. We also evaluate the performance on real artefact cases to showcase the performance of our method. There are two major contributions of this work. First, we address the problem of motion artefact correction directly from k-space by leveraging the rich information available and validate it on a large-scale CMR dataset. Second, we introduce an adverserial component to the Automap framework [18] to increase the realism and quality of the images.

2 Background

Deep learning techniques have been utilized for inverse problems with considerable success [10]. This success has motivated the medical image analysis community to use deep learning on multiple image reconstruction problems such as CT [5] and MR [17]. The main motivation has been to accelerate the image acquisition using under-sampling.

In the literature, there have been four strategies to approach the problem of estimating high quality images from corrupted (or under-sampled) k-space [4]. One choice is to correct the k-space before applying the inverse Fourier transform (IFT). Han et al. [4] proposed the use of convolutional networks for k-space correction coupled with weighting layers on k-space. A more common approach is to use the IFT on k-space and learn a mapping between the corrupted images and good quality images. Kwon et al. [7] proposed using multi-layer preceptrons to find this mapping. This group of approaches are essentially denoising techniques, which do not directly utilize the information in the frequency domain. To remedy this broken link an alternative strategy is to use iterative updates between k-space and the image domain using a cascaded network [14,15]. This group of methods aims to use networks in the image domain to improve the image and feed back the improved image information to k-space with a data consistency term. More recently, Zhu et al. [18] proposed an end-to-end image reconstruction approach (Automap) for MR and evaluated it on under-sampled k-space data.

In the context of CMR artefact correction, early works focused on changes in acquisition schemes [13] and analytical methods for motion artefact reduction [6]. For automatic correction of the CMR, Lotjonen et al. [8] used short-axis and long-axis images to optimize the locations of the slices using mutual information as a similarity measure. However, these methods cannot address the mis-triggering problem and focus only on the in-plane motion of the heart.

3 Methods

The proposed framework of using a deep neural network for motion artefact correction on k-space data is based on a generative-adversarial network setup. Our aim is to train a successful generator to reconstruct good quality images from motion artefact corrupted k-space data.

3.1   Network Architecture

The algorithm consists of a generator and a discriminator as illustrated in Fig. 2. Our generator network follows a similar architecture to [18], which was originally developed for image reconstruction using domain specific information. In our case we additionally use a discriminator to increase the robustness and realism of the reconstructed images. The input to the network is a complex n-by-n k-space matrix, which we concatenate into a $(2 \times n \times n)$-by-1 vector. We then use two fully connected layers: FC1 with $2 \times n \times n$ neurons and FC2 with $n \times n$ neurons. The output from FC2 is reshaped and two convolutional layers with 64 filters and 5×5 filter size are used. After that a deconvolutional layer with 64 filters of size 7×7 is applied and finally a 1×1 layer is used to aggregate the results into an image.

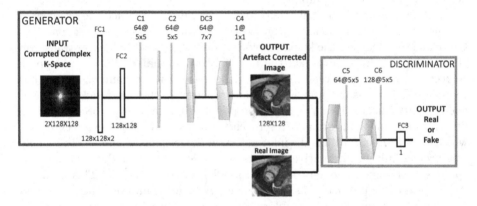

Fig. 2. Generative adversarial Automap architecture for motion artefact correction.

The discriminator takes a generated image or a real image as input and uses two convolutional layers and a final dense layer for classification. The final output of the discriminator a decision as to whether the generated image looks real or fake. By using outputs of the generator (artefact corrected images) and the real images from the dataset the discriminator is trained to distinguish between the artefact corrected images and high quality images. The loss function for the model is a mean squared error loss between the predicted image and real image and combined with a Wasserstein loss [3], which takes the mean of the differences between the two images. The weights of the discriminator are frozen during the training of the whole model and trained separately only with the Wasserstein loss, which is shown to be effective for inverse problems [1].

3.2   Implementation Details

The parameters of the convolutional and fully-connected layers were initialized randomly from a zero-mean Gaussian distribution and trained until no substantial progress was observed in the training loss. In this study, we use the RMSprop optimizer to minimize mean squared error. One important aspect during training is the activity regularizer, which is used after the deconvolutional layer. In our implementation, we first trained without this regularizer, finding that including it early in training led to the loss being trapped in poor local minima. Once training converged without the regularizer, it was then added, which led to the generation of sharper looking images.

First, we trained our network data from the ImageNET dataset to learn a variety of frequencies from k-space as described in [18] without the regularization term. Then, the network was trained for 50 epochs with the regularization term. Finally, we introduced the cardiac MR data and trained our network for an additional 150 epochs. The training was stopped early if no significant improvement was observed. An improvement was considered significant if the relative increase in performance was at least 0.5% over 20 epochs. To better generalize the model we applied data augmentation by rotating images in increments of 90°. We also found that the success of our implementation was highly sensitive to the choice of learning rate, which we set to be 0.00002.

During training, a batch-size of 20 2D k-space datasets was used. We used the Keras Framework with Tensorflow backend for implementation and training the network took around 3 days on a NVIDIA Quadro 6000P GPU. Correction of a single image sequence took less than 1s once the network was trained.

4   Experimental Results

We evaluated our algorithm on a subset of the UK Biobank dataset consisting of 2000 good quality CINE MR acquisitions. 50 temporal frames from each subject at mid-ventricular level were used to generate synthetic motion artefacts. We used 75000 2D images for training and 25000 images for testing. The data were chosen to be free of other types of image quality issues such as missing axial slices and were visually verified by an expert cardiologist. The details of the acquisition protocol of the UK Biobank dataset can be found in [12].

4.1   K-space Corruption for Synthetic Data

We generated k-space corrupted data in order to simulate motion artefacts. We followed a Cartesian sampling strategy for k-space corruption to generate synthetic but realistic motion artefacts [11]. We first transformed each 2D short axis sequence to the Fourier domain and changed 1 in 3 Cartesian sampling lines to the corresponding lines from other cardiac phases to mimic motion artefacts. We added a random frame offset when replacing the lines. In this way the original good quality images from the training set were used to generate corresponding CMR artefact images. This is a realistic approach as the motion artefacts that occur from mis-triggering often arise from similar misplacement of k-space lines.

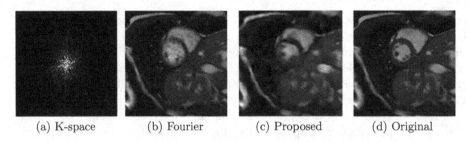

(a) K-space   (b) Fourier   (c) Proposed   (d) Original

Fig. 3. Synthetic dataset results. Corrupted k-space (a), inverse Fourier transform (b), proposed method (c) and original good quality image (d). The proposed method is able to correct the motion artefacts, but loses some structure.

4.2 Quantitative Results on Synthetic Dataset

We compared our algorithm with a reconstruction using the IFT and also with two variants of the proposed deep learning framework: one without the adversarial component and one with the adversarial component but trained only using ImageNET data. The results are reported in Table 1. We report root mean square error (RMSE) and peak signal-to-noise ratio (PSNR) results for motion artefact correction, defined as follows:

$$\text{RMSE} = \sqrt{\frac{1}{N_x N_y} \sum_{x=0}^{N_x} \sum_{y=0}^{N_y} (r(x,y) - p(x,y))^2}$$

$$\text{PSNR} = 20 log_{10} \left(\frac{\sum_{x=0}^{N_x} \sum_{y=0}^{N_y} r(x,y)^2}{\sqrt{\sum_{x=0}^{N_x} \sum_{y=0}^{N_y} (r(x,y) - p(x,y))^2}} \right)$$

where N_x and N_y denote the number of pixels in the x and y directions and r and p represent reference and predicted images.

Alongside these two measures, we also computed structural similarity index (SSIM) [16] results. SSIM has been shown to provide sensitivity to structural information and texture. The SSIM between two images is defined as follows for any image region x and y:

$$\text{SSIM}(x,y) = \frac{(2\mu_x\mu_y + c_1)(2\sigma_{xy} + c_2)}{(\mu_x^2 + \mu_y^2 + c_1)(\sigma_x^2 + \sigma_y^2 + c_2)}$$

where μ_x and μ_y are the average intensities for regions x and y, σ_x and σ_y are variance values for regions x and y, σ_{xy} is the covariance of regions x and y and c_1 and c_2 are constant values for stabilizing the denominator.

Table 1 shows that the cardiac trained adversarial Automap technique is capable of correcting motion artefacts with high accuracy compared to the other techniques. The quality of the images increased particularly in terms of low RMSE and high PSNR using the ImageNET trained Automap reconstruction compared to the IFT reconstruction approach. However, some structure has been lost in comparison with the IFT approach, which can be seen from the lower SSIM scores with the proposed method. Training with cardiac images helped to recover some SSIM, but it was still lower than the IFT approach. One possible explanation for this is that in the proposed method, the network has been trained to minimise the MSE, which commonly causes smoothed-out or blurred looking images. An example of such a case can be seen in Fig. 3, where the proposed method corrects the artefact but loses some structural information. The adversarial training improves the performance of the Automap model in all three metrics and especially in terms of SSIM.

Table 1. Mean RMSE, PSNR, and SSIM results of motion artefact correction from k-space data.

Methods	RMSE	PSNR	SSIM
Inverse Fourier Transform	0.045	27.8	**0.883**
Proposed-ImageNET	0.032	31.1	0.766
Automap-Cardiac [18]	0.029	32.7	0.814
Proposed-Cardiac	**0.027**	**35.1**	0.850

4.3 Qualitative Results on Real Motion Artefact Case

To illustrate the performance of our technique on artefact correction, we applied it to a dataset from the UK Biobank containing mis-triggering artefacts. The visual results in Fig. 4 show improved image quality compared to the IFT reconstructed image.

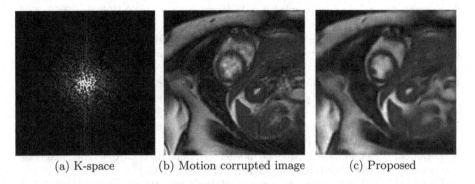

(a) K-space   (b) Motion corrupted image   (c) Proposed

Fig. 4. Example of a mis-triggering artefact from the UK Biobank dataset. K-space data (a), motion corrupted image (b) and proposed method (c). The proposed method is able to correct the motion artefacts.

5   Discussion and Conclusion

In this paper, we have proposed an end-to-end image artefact correction pipeline for 2D CINE CMR, and evaluated it on the large-scale UK Biobank dataset. We have shown the value and shortcomings of deep learning based reconstruction for motion artefact correction. We have demonstrated that the generic Automap framework can aid in correcting motion artefacts using an adversarial setup, outperforming inverse Fourier transform. To the best knowledge of the authors, this is the first paper that has addressed the motion artefact correction problem in MR directly from k-space data. The general applicability of the Automap framework is limited by its high memory requirement, which is caused by the fully connected layers at the start of the network.

In future work, we plan to investigate more appropriate loss functions to attempt to recover the lost structural information in the reconstructed images. Moreover, we will investigate the robustness of our technique on our own clinical data, which we expect to contain more motion corruption compared to UK Biobank data.

Acknowledgments. This work was supported by an EPSRC programme Grant (EP/P001009/1) and the Wellcome EPSRC Centre for Medical Engineering at the School of Biomedical Engineering and Imaging Sciences, King's College London (WT 203148/Z/16/Z). This research has been conducted using the UK Biobank Resource under Application Number 17806. The GPU used in this research was generously donated by the NVIDIA Corporation.

References

1. Adler, J., et al.: Learning to solve inverse problems using Wasserstein loss. arXiv:1710.10898 (2017)
2. Ferreira, P.F., et al.: Cardiovascular magnetic resonance artefacts. JCMR **15**, 1–41 (2013)
3. Frogner, C., et al.: Learning with a Wasserstein loss. In: NIPS, pp. 2053–2061 (2015)
4. Han, Y., et al.: k-Space deep learning for accelerated MRI. arXiv:1805.03779 (2018)
5. Jin, K.H., et al.: Deep convolutional neural network for inverse problems in imaging. IEEE TIP **26**(9), 4509–4522 (2017)
6. Kim, Y.C., et al.: Automatic correction of echoplanar imaging (EPI) ghosting artifacts in realtime interactive cardiac MRI using sensitivity encoding. JMRI **27**(1), 239–245 (2008)
7. Kwon, K., et al.: A parallel MR imaging method using multilayer perceptron. Med. Phys. **44**(12), 6209–6224 (2017)
8. Lotjonen, J., et al.: Correction of motion artifacts from cardiac cine magnetic resonance images. Acad. Radiol. **12**(10), 1273–1284 (2005)
9. Lustig, M., et al.: Compressed sensing MRI. IEEE Sig. Process. Mag. **25**(2), 72–82 (2008)
10. McCann, M.T., et al.: Convolutional neural networks for inverse problems in imaging: a review. IEEE Sig. Process. Mag. **34**(6), 85–95 (2017)

11. Oksuz, I., et al.: Deep learning using K-space based data augmentation for automated cardiac MR motion artefact detection. In: MICCAI (2018)
12. Petersen, S.E., et al.: UK Biobank's cardiovascular magnetic resonance protocol. JCMR **18**(1), 1–8 (2016)
13. Saremi, F., et al.: Optimizing cardiac MR imaging: practical remedies for artifacts. Radiographics **28**(4), 1161–1187 (2008)
14. Schlemper, J., et al.: A deep cascade of convolutional neural networks for MR image reconstruction. In: IPMI (2017)
15. Schlemper, J., et al.: A deep cascade of convolutional neural networks for dynamic MR image reconstruction. IEEE TMI **37**(2), 491–503 (2018)
16. Wang, Z., et al.: Image quality assessment: from error visibility to structural similarity. IEEE TIP **13**(4), 600–612 (2004)
17. Yang, G., et al.: DAGAN: deep de-aliasing generative adversarial networks for fast compressed sensing MRI reconstruction. IEEE TMI **37**, 1310–1321 (2017)
18. Zhu, B., et al.: Image reconstruction by domain-transform manifold learning. Nature **555**(7697), 487 (2018)

Complex Fully Convolutional Neural Networks for MR Image Reconstruction

Muneer Ahmad Dedmari[1,2(✉)], Sailesh Conjeti[1,2], Santiago Estrada[1,2],
Phillip Ehses[1], Tony Stöcker[1], and Martin Reuter[1,3]

[1] German Center for Neurodegenrative Diseases (DZNE), Bonn, Germany
dedmari_muneer@tum.de
[2] Computer Aided Medical Procedures, Technische Universität München, Munich,
Germany
[3] Harvard University and Massachusetts General Hospital, Boston, USA

Abstract. Undersampling the k-space data is widely adopted for acceleration of Magnetic Resonance Imaging (MRI). Current deep learning based approaches for supervised learning of MRI image reconstruction employ real-valued operations and representations by treating complex valued k-space/spatial-space as real values. In this paper, we propose complex dense fully convolutional neural network ($\mathbb{C}$DFNet) for learning to de-alias the reconstruction artifacts within undersampled MRI images. We fashioned a densely-connected fully convolutional block tailored for complex-valued inputs by introducing dedicated layers such as complex convolution, batch normalization, non-linearities *etc.* $\mathbb{C}$DFNet leverages the inherently complex-valued nature of input k-space and learns richer representations. We demonstrate improved perceptual quality and recovery of anatomical structures through $\mathbb{C}$DFNet in contrast to its real-valued counterparts.

1 Introduction

Magnetic Resonance (MR) Imaging is widely adopted in many diagnostic applications due to its improved soft-tissue contrast, non-invasiveness and excellent spatial resolution. However, MRI is associated with long scan durations as the data is read out sequentially in k-space and the speed at which the k-space can be traversed is limited by the underlying imaging physics. This in turn limits the clinical use of MRI, causes inconvenience to patients, and renders this modality expensive and less accessible. One potential approach to accelerate MRI acquisition is to undersample k-space *i.e.* reduce the number of k-space traversals made during acquisition. However, such an undersampling violates the Nyquist-Shannon Sampling theorem [7] and generates aliasing artefacts upon reconstruction. A learning based reconstruction algorithm should effectively compensate for missing k-space samples by leveraging *a priori* knowledge of the anatomy at hand and the undersampling pattern.

Deep learning is being increasingly adopted for MR reconstruction. Instead of using handcrafted features, Hammernik *et al.* [4] demonstrated learning a set

© Springer Nature Switzerland AG 2018
F. Knoll et al. (Eds.): MLMIR 2018, LNCS 11074, pp. 30–38, 2018.
https://doi.org/10.1007/978-3-030-00129-2_4

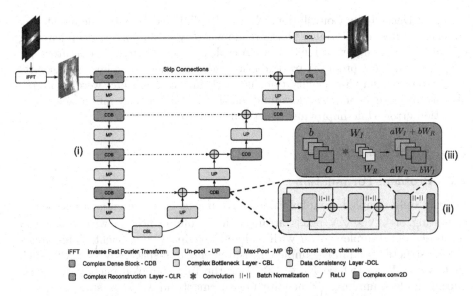

Fig. 1. (i) Complex fully convolutional neural network architecture. (ii) Complex dense block, composed of 3 complex conv2D layers, followed by complex batch normalization and ReLU. (iii) Complex Conv2D layer, responsible for performing complex convolution operation, here a and b represents real and complex feature maps, and W_R and W_I represents real and imaginary parts of learnable weights.

of regularizers under a variational framework, for reconstruction of accelerated MRI data. Kinam *et al.* [5] used the multilayer perceptron for accelerated parallel MRI. These works were further extended using techniques such as, deep residual learning [6], domain adaptation [13], data consistency layer [10], manifold approximation (AUTOMAP) [14], to name a few. However, all of the above mentioned reconstruction methods employ real-valued convolution operations in the spatial-domain by treating real (amplitude) and imaginary (phase) parts as two independent components. It should be noted that unlike multi-channel images (such as RGB images) where individual channels are acquired independently, MR data is inherently complex-valued in nature. Quadrature detection is employed to measure the changing circularly polarized magnetic field within the scanner which results in two simultaneously acquired data streams with a $\pi/2$ phase difference. Upon digitization, these signals constitute the real and imaginary parts of each complex data point in the k-space. The magnitude derived from this complex valued data mainly carries information about proton density as well as relaxation properties of the tissue. The phase can be used to obtain the information, for example, about magnetic susceptibility, flow, or temperature. To faithfully recover the complete k-space, it is important to learn the co-relationship between these data-streams.

In this paper, for the first time, we explore end-to-end learning with complex-valued data targeted at MR reconstruction. Towards this, we propose the

Complex Dense Fully Convolutional Network (ℂDFNet) by introducing densely connected fully convolutional blocks made with layers supporting deep learning operations on complex valued data. Complex-valued arithmetic operators for deep learning were proposed by Trabelsi *et al.* [11] where complex counterparts of convolution, batch-normalization, network initialization *etc.* were explored. We also propose a composite loss function that simultaneously minimizes reconstruction error while improving structural similarity.

2 Methodology

2.1 Problem Formulation

Let the fully-sampled complex-valued MR image be represented as $\mathbf{x}_f \in \mathbb{C}^N$ consisting of $\sqrt{N} \times \sqrt{N}$ pixels arranged in a column fashion with each pixel composed of a complex vector with real and imaginary components. This image is reconstructed from fully-sampled measurements in k-space, say $\mathbf{y}_f \in \mathbb{C}^N$, such that: $\mathbf{y}_f = \mathbf{F}_f \mathbf{x}_f$, where $\mathbf{F}_f \in \mathbb{C}^{N \times N}$ is the fully sampled encoding matrix. During under-sampling, we acquire measurements in k-space, say $\mathbf{y}_u \in \mathbb{C}^M$ where $M \ll N$. Let the image reconstructed from zero-filling $\mathbf{y}_u$ be represented as $\mathbf{x}_u$, such that $\mathbf{x}_u = \mathbf{F}_u^{-1} \mathbf{y}_u$. Reconstructing $\mathbf{x}_f$ directly from $\mathbf{y}_u$ is ill-posed and direct inversion is not possible due to the under-determined nature of the system of equations. In our approach, we enforce $\mathbf{x}_f$ to be approximated using a complex fully convolutional neural network (represented as $f_\mathbb{C}$). As $\mathbf{x}_u$ is highly-aliased due to sub-Nyquist sampling, $f_\mathbb{C}$ aims at recovering image $\mathbf{x}_\mathbf{r}$ that is as close as possible to an ideal fully sampled image $\mathbf{x}_f$.

2.2 Network Architecture

Complex Dense Block: The densely connected block proposed in [2], introduces feed-forward connections from each layer to every other layer (illustrated in Fig. 1(ii)). Such an architecture choice was demonstrated to encourage feature reusability and strengthen information propagation through the network. We suitably adapt this block for complex valued data by proposing counterparts of classic deep learning layers such as convolution, batch normalization, non-linearity (ReLU), up-sampling *etc.* For sake of brevity, we delve only into the complex convolution (denoted as $*_\mathbb{C}$) in detail. Let $\mathbf{h} = \mathbf{a} + i\mathbf{b}$ be the complex-valued input to convolution layer with weights $\mathbf{W} = \mathbf{W_R} + i\mathbf{W_I}$, the complex convolution between $\mathbf{h}$ and $\mathbf{W}$ is simulated using real-valued arithmetic as: $\mathbf{W} *_\mathbb{C} \mathbf{h} = (\mathbf{a} * \mathbf{W_R} - \mathbf{b} * \mathbf{W_I}) + i(\mathbf{a} * \mathbf{W_I} + \mathbf{b} * \mathbf{W_R})$, as shown in Fig. 1(iii). The complex output feature maps are fed into the complex batch normalization layer, which normalizes the data to have equal variance along the real and imaginary components, thereby ensuring a co-relationship between them. The complex variant of non-linearity ReLU and max-pooling are applied on the real and imaginary channels separately.

Complex Dense Fully Convolutional Network (ℂDFNet): The ℂDFNet $f_\mathbb{C}$ is based on the DenseNet [2] architecture, comprising of a sequence of four densely-connected complex encoder blocks with corresponding densely-connected complex decoder blocks separated by a bottleneck layer (illustrated in Fig. 1(i). The output of the last decoder block is given to a reconstruction layer (with complex convolution operators) for reconstructing the image. The encoders and decoders are stacked and trained in a progressive way $i.e.$ output from one block is used as input to other block. Skip connections are included in the architecture between encoder and corresponding decoder blocks to fuse high-level representations (decoder) with low-level features (encoder) for preserving contextual information. Furthermore, skip connections prevent the vanishing gradient problem, by directly propagating gradients from decoder to respective encoder block. The network $f_{\mathbb{C}}$ takes complex-valued aliased image $\mathbf{x}_u$ (generated by zero-filling under-sampled k-space data $\mathbf{y}_u$) as input to an intermediate reconstructed image $\tilde{\mathbf{x}}_r$ which is fed further into the data consistency layer for imputing missing k-space values.

Data Consistency Layer (DCL): We recover a full reconstructed k-space spectrum $\tilde{\mathbf{y}}_r$ via a Fourier transform on the reconstructed image $\tilde{\mathbf{x}}_r$. To retain all the a $priori$ available k-space values $\mathbf{y}_u$ (collected at spatial locations denoted via mask Ω) and impute only the missing values at locations ($\notin \Omega$), the data consistency layer performs the following operation:

$$\mathbf{y}_r(z) = \begin{cases} \mathbf{y}_u(z) & z \in \Omega \\ \tilde{\mathbf{y}}_r(z) & z \notin \Omega \end{cases} \tag{1}$$

After the DCL layer, the final de-aliased image $\mathbf{x}_r$ is recovered through inverse Fourier transform of $\mathbf{y}_r$. It must be noted that the inclusion of the DCL layer within $f_{\mathbb{C}}$ ensures improved efficacy of the network by focusing exclusively on missing k-space values and enforces consistency with a $priori$ acquired data $\mathbf{y}_u$. Further, the DCL layer does not have any learnable parameters and does not increase the complexity of the network.

2.3   Model Learning and Optimization

The network $f_{\mathbb{C}}$ is optimized to recover missing k-space data while simultaneously preserving fine-grained anatomical details. We adopt a supervised learning approach wherein a training dataset $\mathcal{D}$ of input-target (under-sampled and fully-sampled) pairs $(\mathbf{x}_u, \mathbf{x}_f)$ to train $f_{\mathbb{C}}$. We use a composite loss function comprising of two contributing terms, firstly a mean-squared error term $(\mathcal{L}_{L_2})$ and secondly Structural Similarity Index Measure (SSIM) $(\mathcal{L}_{\text{SSIM}})$ as discussed below:

$\mathcal{L}_{L_2}$ **Loss:** This loss is used to minimize the difference between the reconstructed image $\mathbf{x}_r$ and target fully sampled image $\mathbf{x}_f$.

$$\mathcal{L}_{L_2} = \sum_{(\mathbf{x}_u, \mathbf{x}_f) \in \mathcal{D}} \|\mathbf{x}_f - \mathbf{x}_r\|_2^2 = \sum_{(\mathbf{x}_u, \mathbf{x}_f) \in \mathcal{D}} \|\mathbf{x}_f - f_{\mathbb{C}}(\mathbf{x}_u | \theta)\|_2^2 \tag{2}$$

The $\mathcal{L}_2$ loss penalizes large errors, but fails to capture finer details which the human visual system is sensitive to such as contrast, luminance and structure.

To offset the above shortcoming of $\mathcal{L}_2$ loss, we use SSIM [12], which is perceptually closer to the human visual system, as an additional loss $\mathcal{L}_{\mathrm{SSIM}}$, defined as:

$$\mathcal{L}_{\mathrm{SSIM}} = \sum_{(\mathbf{x}_u, \mathbf{x}_f) \in \mathcal{D}} (1 - \mathcal{S}(\mathbf{x}_r, \mathbf{x}_f)) \tag{3}$$

where $\mathcal{S}(\mathbf{x}_r, \mathbf{x}_f)$ is the SSIM calculated between $\mathbf{x}_r$ and $\mathbf{x}_f$. The composite loss function $\mathcal{L}$ for optimizing f_C is defined as: $\mathcal{L}(\mathbf{x}, f_C(\mathbf{x}_u|\theta)) = \mathcal{L}_{L_2} + \lambda \mathcal{L}_{\mathrm{SSIM}}$, where λ is a scaling constant.

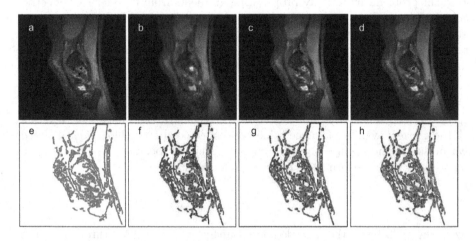

Fig. 2. Edge-map results comparison at undersampling factor of x4. (a), (e) ground-truth and its edge-map, (b), (f) undersampled, and its edge-map (c), (g) DLMRI reconstruction and its edge-map (d), (h) proposed reconstruction and its edge-map. Here, green represents edges present in ground-truth, red represents edges that are missing in reconstructed image, as compared to ground-truth and blue represents edges that are not present in ground-truth but only in reconstructed images. (Color figure online)

3   Results and Discussion

3.1   Experimental Settings and Evaluation

Dataset. Our experiments were evaluated on the publicly available 20 fully-sampled knee k-space dataset from mridata.org [9]. The data was split randomly into 16 patients for training and rest for testing. The coils were fused using sum of squares into a single complete k-space dataset and training data for proof-of-concept was generated using Cartesian under-sampling proposed in [10], wherein eight lowest spatial frequencies were preserved and a zero-mean Gaussian distribution was used to determine the sampling probability along the phase encoding direction (the frequency-encoding direction was fully-sampled).

Baselines and Comparative Methods: To ablatively test the introduction of complex convolution, we compare with the naïve variant of densely connected networks treating the complex-valued input as two independent channels (termed BL1). We further compare the contribution of the data-consistency layer by defining a variant sans DCL (termed BL2). Finally, to evaluate the contribution of training with $\mathcal{L}_{SSIM}$, we set the corresponding factor λ to 0 and contrast with the proposed method (termed BL3). Further, we compare against a state-of-the art dictionary learning based MR reconstruction method proposed in [8] (termed as DLMRI). It must be noted that BL1 is akin to deep learning based reconstruction method proposed in [3], differing only in the usage of densely-connected blocks. In all the aforementioned network configurations, we used complex convolution operators (except BL1) with a depth of 32, and kernel size of 3×3, BL1 was designed with depth of 46 for a fair comparison. Parameters were chosen in such a manner so that model complexity across all baselines remain similar. The networks were trained until convergence using RMSProp as an optimizer with a learning rate of $5e^{-5}$ with decay of 0.9 and batch-size of 5 for 50 epochs.

The networks were evaluated at two acceleration factors of $4\times$ and $6\times$ along the phase-encoding directions. During training of the deep networks, the under-sampling masks were generated on-the-fly to induce the tolerance towards a range of potential aliasing artefacts. We further used image-level rigid and elastic transformations to augment the training data. As demonstrated in [10], fidelity of image reconstruction is evaluated by measuring the similarity between a recon-structed image to the fully-sampled ground truth image using metrics such as SSIM, mean squared error (MSE) *etc.* However, these metrics do not explicitly focus on finer details of the reconstruction and towards this we employ Pratt's figure of merit (Pratt's FOM) [1] as an additional metric. Pratt's FOM exclu-sively focuses on the edges and corner points present in the reconstructed image that are concurrent with structures present in the ground truth image while simultaneously penalizing both missing and artificially hallucinated edges.

3.2   Results

The networks trained for $4\times$ and $6\times$ acceleration factors were tested across and within these factors resulting in four train-test combinations. All the methods were evaluated for each of these combinations to quantify their generalizability to unseen aliasing effects.

Table 1. Pratt's Figure of Merit of comparative analysis against baselines

Acceleration		Pratt's FOM			
Train	Test	BL1	BL2	BL3	Proposed
$4\times$	$4\times$	0.81657	0.77522	0.82480	**0.84364**
$6\times$	$4\times$	0.83961	0.7743	0.82409	**0.84218**
$4\times$	$6\times$	0.71775	0.70099	0.75155	**0.77449**
$6\times$	$6\times$	0.76009	0.7199	0.75661	**0.77514**

BL1: DenseNet with $\lambda = 2$ with DCL
BL2: CDFNet with $\lambda = 2$ without DCL
BL3: CDFNet with $\lambda = 0$ with DCL

Table 2. Quantitative comparison from Cartesian trajectory with undersampling factor of 4× and 6×

Acceleration		SSIM			MSE (x 10^{-4})			Pratt's FOM		
Train	Test	x_u	DLMRI	Proposed	x_u	DLMRI	Proposed	x_u	DLMRI	Proposed
4×	4×	0.8886	0.9173	**0.9269**	11.89	7.01	**5.54**	0.63795	0.73876	**0.84364**
6×	4×			0.9266			5.57			0.84218
4×	6×	0.8552	0.8920	0.9062	17.55	10.70	7.76	0.51309	0.64529	0.77449
6×	6×			**0.9072**			**7.54**			**0.77514**

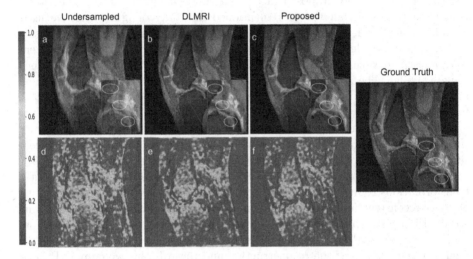

Fig. 3. Reconstruction results using 4× acceleration factor. (a), (d) Undersampled image and its error map, (b), (e) DLMRI reconstruction and its error map, (c), (f) Proposed reconstruction and its error-map, and ground truth.

Qualitative Analysis: Figure 2 illustrates the contrastive results on recovery of fine-grained details using the edge-map extracted from an under-sampled image (Fig. 2(b, f)), DLMRI (Fig. 2(c, g)) and proposed method (Fig. 2(d, h)). We observe that the proposed network demonstrates maximal consistency in finer details with respect to the ground-truth. Figure 3 highlights the differences with respect to the ground truth through a difference map and particularly focus on reconstruction of fine details in the region between the tibia and femur and the synovial membrane.

Ablative Testing: To ablatively evaluate the contributions of this work, the proposed method was contrasted against baselines (discussed in Sect. 3.1) and observations are tabulated in Table 1. For sake of brevity, we only present the Pratt's FOM metric in this table. Contrasting the proposed method against BL1 in Table 1, we observe a consistent improvement in the reconstruction error due to the introduction of complex dense blocks in place of vanilla dense blocks. This is particularly evident for the case of aggressive under-sampling ($6\times$) where the proposed method outperformed BL1 with a significant margin of 5.7%. Comparing BL2 with the proposed method, the inclusion of the data consistency layer proved to be of high significance as evidenced across all validation combinations with an average improvement of over 6%. The use of SSIM as an additional loss function during optimization (comparing BL3 with proposed method) also consistently improves Pratt's FOM across all the test cases.

Comparative Methods: In Table 2, we compare the proposed method against the under-sampled input image (x_u) and state-of-art compressed sensing approach, DLMRI, in terms of the evaluation metrics SSIM, MSE and Pratt's FOM. We observe consistent improvement across all metrics in comparison to DLMRI, with the proposed method being able to recover finer details significantly (over 11% improvement in Pratt's FOM). In scenarios of testing on aggressive acceleration ($6\times$), which corresponds to the limit of sparsity based methods, we observe that CDFNet recovers anatomical details better as it is learnt in an end-to-end fashion allowing for efficient learning of anatomical priors from the training data.

4   Conclusion and Future Work

We have presented a deep learning based MR imaging reconstruction method, wherein real-valued neural network operations are replaced by complex convolutional operations. In this work, we demonstrated that the proposed network architecture outperformed the standard state-of art and the real-valued counter part methods by significant margins in terms of recovering fine structures and high frequency textures. The experiments also show that the proposed method is robust towards the undersampling ratio, which eliminates the need for training multiple large networks for each acquisition settings. Finally, Pratt's figure of merit was adapted for performing evaluation by considering the overall perceptual quality of reconstructed image. As k-space is inherently complex-valued, we believe that this method can be adapted to learn both, domain transformation as well as reconstruction. Moreover, non-Cartesian trajectories can be investigated, as they possess different aliasing properties, a further validation is appropriate to determine the flexibility of our method towards this end.

References

1. Hagara, M., Hlavatovic, A.: Video segmentation based on Pratt's figure of merit. In: 2009 19th International Conference Radioelektronika, pp. 91–94, April 2009. https://doi.org/10.1109/RADIOELEK.2009.5158758
2. Huang, G., Liu, Z., Weinberger, K.Q.: Densely connected convolutional networks. CoRR abs/1608.06993 (2016)
3. Hyun, C.M., Kim, H.P., Lee, S.M., Lee, S., Seo, J.K.: Deep learning for undersampled MRI reconstruction. Phys. Med. Biol. (2018)

4. Hammernik, K., et al.: Learning a variational network for reconstruction of accelerated MRI data. Magn. Resonance Med. **79**(6), 3055–3071 (2018)
5. Kinam, K., Dongchan, K., HyunWook, P.: A parallel MR imaging method using multilayer perceptron. Med. Phys. **44**(12), 6209–6224 (2017)
6. Lee, D., Yoo, J.J., Tak, S., Ye, J.C.: Deep residual learning for accelerated MRI using magnitude and phase networks. CoRR abs/1804.00432 (2018)
7. Nyquist, H.: Certain topics in telegraph transmission theory. Trans. Am. Inst. Electr. Eng. **47**(2), 617–644 (1928)
8. Ravishankar, S., Bresler, Y.: MR image reconstruction from highly undersampled k-space data by dictionary learning. IEEE Trans. Med. Imaging **30**(5), 1028–1041 (2011)
9. Sawyer, A.M., et al.: Creation of fully sampled MR data repository for compressed sensing of the knee. Ge Healthcare (2013)
10. Schlemper, J., Caballero, J., Hajnal, J.V., Price, A.N., Rueckert, D.: A deep cascade of convolutional neural networks for MR image reconstruction. CoRR abs/1703.00555 (2017)
11. Trabelsi, C., et al.: Deep complex networks. CoRR abs/1705.09792 (2017)
12. Wang, Z., Bovik, A.C., Sheikh, H.R., Simoncelli, E.P.: Image quality assessment: from error visibility to structural similarity. IEEE Trans. Image Process. **13**(4), 600–612 (2004)
13. Yoseob, H., Jaejun, Y., Hee, K.H., Jung, S.H., Kyunghyun, S., Chul, Y.J.: Deep learning with domain adaptation for accelerated projection reconstruction MR. Magn. Resonance Med. **80**(3), 1189–1205 (2018)
14. Zhu, B., Liu, J.Z., Cauley, S.F., Rosen, B.R., Rosen, M.S.: Image reconstruction by domain-transform manifold learning. Nature **555**, 487 EP (2018)

Magnetic Resonance Fingerprinting Reconstruction via Spatiotemporal Convolutional Neural Networks

Fabian Balsiger[1]([⊠]) [iD], Amaresha Shridhar Konar[2], Shivaprasad Chikop[2],
Vimal Chandran[1], Olivier Scheidegger[3], Sairam Geethanath[2],
and Mauricio Reyes[1]

[1] Institute for Surgical Technology and Biomechanics, University of Bern,
Bern, Switzerland
`fabian.balsiger@istb.unibe.ch`
[2] Medical Imaging Research Center, Dayananda Sagar Institutions, Bangalore, India
[3] Support Center for Advanced Neuroimaging (SCAN),
Institute for Diagnostic and Interventional Neuroradiology, Inselspital,
Bern University Hospital, University of Bern, Bern, Switzerland

Abstract. Magnetic resonance fingerprinting (MRF) quantifies multiple nuclear magnetic resonance parameters in a single and fast acquisition. Standard MRF reconstructs parametric maps using dictionary matching, which lacks scalability due to computational inefficiency. We propose to perform MRF map reconstruction using a spatiotemporal convolutional neural network, which exploits the relationship between neighboring MRF signal evolutions to replace the dictionary matching. We evaluate our method on multiparametric brain scans and compare it to three recent MRF reconstruction approaches. Our method achieves state-of-the-art reconstruction accuracy and yields qualitatively more appealing maps compared to other reconstruction methods. In addition, the reconstruction time is significantly reduced compared to a dictionary-based approach.

Keywords: Magnetic resonance fingerprinting · Parameter mapping
Image reconstruction · Convolutional neural network

1 Introduction

Magnetic resonance imaging (MRI) is widely used in healthcare centers for the diagnosis of pathologies. The diagnosis from MRI relies mostly on weighted images, where the contrast between tissues is used to identify pathologies rather than the absolute intensities in the images. This qualitative approach limits the objective evaluation and reproducibility of MRI in the clinics. Although significant effort has been made for quantitative MRI, a clinical relevant solution for nuclear magnetic resonance (NMR) parameter mapping has not been achieved so far. Mainly time-inefficiency and the limitation to one NMR parameter at

© Springer Nature Switzerland AG 2018
F. Knoll et al. (Eds.): MLMIR 2018, LNCS 11074, pp. 39–46, 2018.
https://doi.org/10.1007/978-3-030-00129-2_5

interest (e.g. T1 and T2 relaxation times) make quantitative MRI inappropriate for clinical use. To overcome the drawbacks of quantitative MRI, magnetic resonance fingerprinting (MRF) has been proposed recently as a novel quantitative MRI technique [6]. MRF quantifies multiple NMR parameters in a single and fast acquisition. The acquisition relies on a MR sequence with pseudo-randomly varying parameters to obtain a unique signal evolution, i.e. fingerprint, per tissue and voxel. After the acquisition, a dictionary matching algorithm assigns the voxel's signal evolutions to an entry of a dictionary of simulated and pre-computed signal evolutions, which allows reconstructing quantitative maps of NMR parameters of interest. However, this dictionary matching is time-consuming, lacks scalability, and can introduce artefacts due to the under-sampled k-space during the acquisition [8].

Recently, three approaches have been proposed aiming to overcome the issues associated with dictionary matching during the MRF reconstruction. Gómez et al. [4] proposed a spatiotemporal dictionary matching that matches a spatial neighborhood of fingerprints instead of using a fingerprint-wise approach. They additionally improve the computational efficiency by limiting the matching to a local search window. However, the search window comes at the cost of requiring spatially aligned MRF scans, and ultimately only alleviates the problem of scalability of dictionary-based MRF reconstruction methods. Therefore, approaches replacing the dictionary matching using deep learning have been proposed to overcome the bottleneck of scalability. Cohen et al. [3] proposed a fully-connected neural network and Hoppe et al. [5] proposed a convolutional neural network (CNN) to learn the matching of a MRF signal evolution to NMR properties. Both approaches show promising results regarding reconstruction accuracy and speed, and their concepts might be a feasible way to replace the dictionary matching involved in MRF reconstruction. However, they use a fingerprint-wise approach, i.e. do not consider any spatial characteristics during the reconstruction, which might result in noisy reconstructions. Moreover, all three approaches use maps reconstructed by the standard dictionary matching with simulated entries as ground truth to compare their reconstructed maps. This ultimately adds a bias to the methods, which resemble the dictionary matching instead of learning the underlying relation of the fingerprints to the NMR parameter maps.

We propose a MRF reconstruction approach that exploits the spatiotemporal relationship between neighboring signal evolutions motivated by noisy reconstructions of fingerprint-wise approaches and the findings of [4]. Our approach bases on CNNs and yields fast and more accurate reconstructions than recently proposed methods on six healthy brain MRF images with three NMR maps: proton density (PD), T1 relaxation time (T1), and T2 relaxation time (T2). Unlike previously published methods, we rely on parametric maps acquired trough MR parameter mapping as ground truth instead of reconstructed maps by dictionary matching. We compare our performance to the aforementioned spatiotemporal dictionary- and deep learning-based methods. We report quantitative and qualitative results and discuss open issues and challenges towards a relevant solution for accurate and fast MRF reconstruction.

2 Materials and Methods

We consider a four-dimensional (4-D) MRF image $I \in \mathbb{C}^{X \times Y \times Z \times T}$, where each voxel $I(\mathbf{v}) = \{t_1, t_2, \ldots, t_T\}$ at location $\mathbf{v} = (x, y, z)$ contains a MRF signal evolution, or fingerprint, with T temporal signal intensities t_i. For each MRF image I, a set $Q = \{q_1, q_2, \ldots, q_M\} \in \mathbb{R}^{X \times Y \times Z \times M}$ with M parametric maps are available as ground truth for the reconstruction. In this work, six brain MRF images with $M = 3$ parametric maps $Q = \{PD, T1, T2\}$ were used.

2.1 MRF and Parametric Map Acquisition

We acquired brain scans from six healthy male volunteers (21 to 43 years) using a tailored MRF sequence [7] on a 1.5 Tesla GE SIGNA Artist scanner (GE Medical Systems, Milwaukee, WI, U.S.) with a 16-channel head coil as part of an institution approved study. Each scan consisted of $Z = 16$ axial-oriented slices with a matrix size of $X \times Y = 256 \times 256$, field of view (FOV) of 256×256 mm^2, voxel size of $1.0 \times 1.0 \times 5.0$ mm^3, and a total of 720 temporal images per slice. After the acquisition, the images were pre-processed using a sliding-window reconstruction [1] with a window size of 48 resulting in $T = 673$ temporal images.

The parametric maps serving as ground truth for the MRF reconstruction were acquired with the same number of slices, matrix size, FOV, and voxel size. The T1 and T2 maps were generated using curve fitting of the MR signal of multi-FA and multi-echo sequences, respectively. Seven T1-weighted images were acquired with a gradient recalled echo pulse sequence with FAs of 1°, 2°, 5°, 8°, 11°, 14°, and 25°, and constant TR/TE = 5.85/1.77 ms. A fast spin echo sequence with eight TEs starting from 20 ms at an interval of 20 ms was used to generate the T2 map (FA = 90° and TR = 1626 ms). By using a signal intensity equation, the PD maps were generated from the T1-weighted images acquired for the T1 mapping.

2.2 Spatiotemporal CNN MRF Reconstruction

We propose a CNN to learn spatiotemporal features to reconstruct the maps Q from a MRF image I. Input to the CNN are MRF image patches $I_P(\mathbf{v}) \in \mathbb{C}^{5 \times 5 \times T} \subset I$, centered at location $\mathbf{v}$. Output of the CNN are the values of the estimated maps $\hat{Q}(\mathbf{v}) \in \mathbb{R}^M$ at location $\mathbf{v}$. The CNN is trained to learn the mapping $\mathcal{M} : I_P(\mathbf{v}) \rightarrow Q(\mathbf{v})$. We remark that the reconstruction was performed slice-wise due to the large slice spacing of 5.0 mm of our data. Figure 1 provides an overview of how the input and output data are defined for the proposed multiparametric spatiotemporal MRF reconstruction.

Pre-processing. We first apply a brain mask to the MRF images and the corresponding maps to exclude the background in all experiments. The masks were manually segmented using the T1 map with the polygon tool in ITK-SNAP

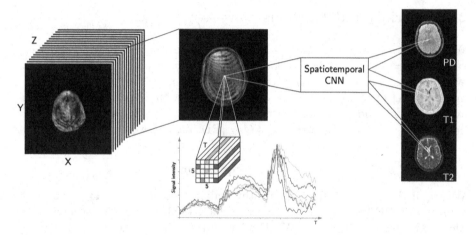

Fig. 1. Overview of the proposed spatiotemporal MRF reconstruction. Note that the signal evolutions are complex-valued but the absolute numbers are plotted for simplicity.

(www.itksnap.org). Outliers from each map in Q are removed by clipping the values to the percentiles $[0.1, 99.9]$. Finally, we normalize I along the temporal axis T to have zero mean and unit variance, and Q along the temporal axis M to the range $[0, 1]$. Note that within each subject the maps were spatially aligned and therefore no registration was applied.

Architecture. Our network consists of five convolutional layers, which learn the mapping $\mathcal{M}$, i.e. we predict the M map values at location $\mathbf{v}$ from an MRF image patch I_P (Fig. 2). We first concatenate the real and imaginary part of the complex-valued input $I_P(\mathbf{v}) \in \mathbb{C}^{5 \times 5 \times T}$ to a real-valued input $I_P(\mathbf{v}) \in \mathbb{R}^{5 \times 5 \times 2T}$ and consider the temporal dimension $(2T)$ as the channels in our network. Second, we apply two 1×1 convolutional blocks to reduce the number of channels to 256. Subsequently, we apply two convolutional blocks in parallel with different receptive fields of 5×5 and 3×3 motivated by [2]. The output channels of these two convolutional blocks are concatenated and fed into the last convolutional layer with M output channels corresponding to the values of the estimated maps $\hat{Q}$. A convolutional block in our network consists of a sequence of 2-D convolutional layer (valid padding and stride one), dropout, batch normalization, and rectified linear unit (ReLU) activation function. We maintain a linear activation at the last convolutional layer (valid padding and stride one). The estimated maps are denormalized to get quantitative values in the range prior to the pre-processing. We implemented our network using the open source machine learning library TensorFlow 1.8.0 (Google, Mountain View, CA, U.S.) with Python 3.6 (Python Software Foundation, Wilmington, DE, U.S.).

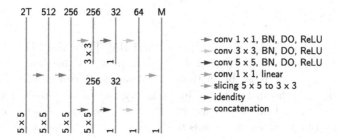

Fig. 2. The architecture of our spatiotemporal CNN. To perform a convolution with a filter size of 3 × 3, we extract a 3 × 3 patch from a 5 × 5 patch denoted as slicing operation. The number of channels are denoted on the top of the bars and the $x \times y$ size is provided at the lower left edge of the bars. BN: batch normalization, DO: dropout.

Training. The network was trained using an Adam optimizer with a learning rate of 0.001, which minimized a mean squared error (MSE) loss with a batch size of 600 randomly sampled patches I_P. The dropout rate was set to 0.2 and the training was stopped after 50 epochs, which we empirically found to be sufficient.

2.3 Evaluation

We evaluate the performance our model and the baselines using a leave-one-out cross-validation, i.e. we train the model on five brain scans and test it on the left-out brain scan. Note that we tuned the architecture on one randomly chosen cross-validation split and did not use the other splits to develop and tune the architecture.

Baselines. We compare our method to recent approaches for MRF reconstruction using the fully-connected neural network [3], the CNN [5], and the spatiotemporal dictionary matching [4]. For the deep learning-based methods, we performed the same leave-one-out cross-validation and the data underwent the same pre-processing as for our method. The approaches were implemented as proposed in the papers. For [4], we also perform a leave-one-out cross-validation, i.e. construct a dictionary using five brain scans and reconstruct the left-out brain scan with following parameters: $W_n = 11 \times 11 \times 3$, $P = 3 \times 3 \times 3$, $C = 5$, and $\alpha = 0.5$ with two iterations.

Metrics. Quantitatively, we report the mean and standard deviation of the mean absolute difference (MAE) and the root mean square error (RMSE) for the leave-one-out cross-validation. The metrics are reported separately for the three brain tissues white matter (WM), gray matter (GM), and cerebrospinal fluid (CSF). The brain tissue masks were obtained from the T1 maps using thresholding according to literature values [6].

3   Results

Mean and standard deviation of the MAE and RMSE for the PD, T1, and T2 map reconstructions are given in Table 1. The proposed method outperforms the other methods for most brain tissues and maps. Reconstructed maps of a mid-brain slice are shown in Fig. 3. Qualitatively, our maps show a good reconstruction with visible brain structures like the ventricles. It is noticeable that our spatiotemporal approach yields a less noisy reconstruction than the fingerprint-wise approach of Cohen et al. [3] (similar noisy reconstructions were obtained for Hoppe et al. [5] but not reported in Fig. 3). The dictionary-based approach [4] yields a qualitatively coarser reconstruction than our method. Overall, large reconstruction errors are mainly present at the skull, meninges, ventricles as well as at the boundary of the brain mask (rightmost column in Fig. 3), which could be consistently observed for all methods.

Table 1. Mean absolute error (MAE) and root mean square error (RMSE) for the PD, T1, and T2 map reconstructions separated by the brain tissues white matter (WM), gray matter (GM), and cerebrospinal fluid (CSF).

Tissue	Method	PD		T1 (ms)		T2 (ms)	
		MAE	RMSE	MAE	RMSE	MAE	RMSE
WM	Cohen	0.084 ± 0.030	0.107 ± 0.032	209.0 ± 28.3	267.5 ± 21.5	43.6 ± 23.9	77.3 ± 54.7
	Hoppe	0.080 ± 0.030	0.101 ± 0.031	253.9 ± 64.3	317.7 ± 67.2	61.3 ± 36.3	92.0 ± 53.8
	Gómez	0.058 ± 0.015	0.074 ± 0.021	258.6 ± 61.0	327.2 ± 68.5	33.4 ± 20.4	73.4 ± 50.6
	Proposed	**0.055 ± 0.015**	**0.072 ± 0.016**	**159.4 ± 36.3**	**242.7 ± 54.7**	**28.0 ± 17.6**	**71.1 ± 62.0**
GM	Cohen	0.094 ± 0.028	0.121 ± 0.026	197.0 ± 28.4	**258.0 ± 42.0**	57.6 ± 35.4	97.3 ± 65.9
	Hoppe	0.092 ± 0.030	0.119 ± 0.029	218.5 ± 37.6	287.5 ± 42.5	70.2 ± 41.0	105.1 ± 61.7
	Gómez	**0.060 ± 0.017**	0.081 ± 0.021	**190.8 ± 24.7**	269.1 ± 43.1	45.8 ± 26.9	**90.5 ± 59.6**
	Proposed	0.061 ± 0.017	**0.077 ± 0.020**	208.2 ± 34.1	286.6 ± 46.5	**43.2 ± 31.2**	93.6 ± 76.3
CSF	Cohen	0.126 ± 0.024	0.152 ± 0.025	1162.6 ± 256.2	1364.1 ± 265.1	183.3 ± 54.1	237.0 ± 58.0
	Hoppe	0.128 ± 0.013	0.156 ± 0.014	1013.3 ± 236.0	1219.4 ± 251.5	**174.7 ± 49.3**	**227.8 ± 55.5**
	Gómez	0.102 ± 0.020	0.129 ± 0.019	1072.5 ± 164.5	1268.8 ± 172.6	228.6 ± 85.7	286.8 ± 86.0
	Proposed	**0.093 ± 0.013**	**0.113 ± 0.009**	**989.2 ± 254.7**	**1181.5 ± 288.6**	181.6 ± 48.6	240.2 ± 48.7

4   Discussion and Conclusion

We presented a deep learning-based, dictionary-free approach to reconstruct parametric maps from MRF images that exploits the spatiotemporal relationship between neighboring fingerprints. The approach is designed as CNN that yields a reconstruction of parametric maps in a more accurate way than previously proposed dictionary-free methods and competes with a dictionary-based method.

In general, the results show that a spatiotemporal reconstruction is favorable to a fingerprint-wise reconstruction for almost all brain tissues and parametric maps (Table 1). Out of the three brain tissues, the GM yielded the most inconsistent results among the different methods. We think that this might arise due to partial volume effects at the interface to WM and CSF. A spatial analysis reveals high reconstruction errors in the skull, meningeal layers, and ventricles for all

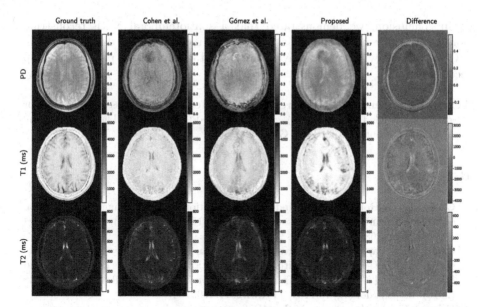

Fig. 3. Exemplary map reconstructions of one axial brain slice. The rows represent the three maps PD, T1, and T2. The columns represent from left to right: the ground truth map, results of Cohen et al. [3], Gómez et al. [4], and our proposed method. The rightmost column shows the difference $\hat{Q} - Q$ between our estimated map $\hat{Q}$ and the ground truth map Q.

methods (rightmost column in Fig. 3). These reconstruction errors could origin from a partial volume effect or an apparent lack of training examples. Reconstruction artifacts are only present in the method of Gómez et al. [4], confirming the findings of [8]. In regards to the computational costs, all deep learning-based approaches yield reconstructed maps within few seconds. Conversely, the dictionary-based approach is computationally intensive, with calculations in the order of several minutes per reconstruction. For clinically used MRF reconstruction, we therefore think that machine learning-based approaches are favorable to dictionary-based approaches in the long term.

Our study design included parametric maps acquired trough MR parameter mapping as ground truth. The reconstruction errors of all methods are large compared to the errors reported in the studies of the baselines [3–5]. Such large errors are especially surprising for the dictionary-based method, which can be interpreted as a k-nearest neighbor search. Unfortunately, all baselines compared their performance with a ground truth obtained by dictionary matching as proposed in the original MRF paper [6]. Therefore, the methods resembled the dictionary matching instead of learning the underlying relation between fingerprints and NMR maps. We think that a comparison to acquired NMR maps is ultimately more meaningful than a comparison with maps reconstructed from simulated dictionaries. Our results suggest that the direct learning of fingerprints to acquired NMR maps is possible, although additional investigations and work are needed to lower the reconstruction errors.

In conclusion, we demonstrated that a spatiotemporal MRF reconstruction is favorable to a fingerprint-wise MRF reconstruction designed within a CNN by achieving quantitatively and qualitatively better parametric map reconstructions.

Acknowledgements. This research was supported by the Swiss Foundation for Research on Muscle Diseases (ssem), grant attributed to author OS. The authors thank the NVIDIA Corporation for their GPU donation.

References

1. Cao, X., et al.: Robust sliding-window reconstruction for accelerating the acquisition of MR fingerprinting. Magn. Reson. Med. **78**(4), 1579–1588 (2017). https://doi.org/10.1002/mrm.26521
2. Chen, L.C., Papandreou, G., Kokkinos, I., Murphy, K., Yuille, A.L.: DeepLab: semantic image segmentation with deep convolutional nets, atrous convolution, and fully connected CRFs. IEEE Trans. Pattern Anal. Mach. Intell. **40**(4), 834–848 (2016). https://doi.org/10.1109/TPAMI.2017.2699184
3. Cohen, O., Zhu, B., Rosen, M.S.: MR fingerprinting deep reconstruction network (DRONE). Magnetic Reson. Med. **80**(3), 885–894 (2018). https://doi.org/10.1002/mrm.27198
4. Gómez, P.A., et al.: Simultaneous parameter mapping, modality synthesis, and anatomical labeling of the brain with MR fingerprinting. In: Ourselin, S., Joskowicz, L., Sabuncu, M.R., Unal, G., Wells, W. (eds.) MICCAI 2016. LNCS, vol. 9902, pp. 579–586. Springer, Cham (2016). https://doi.org/10.1007/978-3-319-46726-9_67
5. Hoppe, E., et al.: Deep learning for magnetic resonance fingerprinting: a new approach for predicting quantitative parameter values from time series. In: Röhrig, R., Timmer, A., Binder, H., Sax, U. (eds.) German Medical Data Sciences: Visions and Bridges, Oldenburg, vol. 243, pp. 202–206 (2017). https://doi.org/10.3233/978-1-61499-808-2-202
6. Ma, D., et al.: Magnetic resonance fingerprinting. Nature **495**(7440), 187–192 (2013). https://doi.org/10.1038/nature11971
7. Shaik, I., et al.: Tailored magnetic resonance fingerprinting: optimizing acquisition schedule and intelligent reconstruction using a block approach. In: ISMRM 2018 (2018)
8. Wang, Z., Zhang, Q., Yuan, J., Wang, X.: MRF denoising with compressed sensing and adaptive filtering. In: 2014 IEEE 11th International Symposium on Biomedical Imaging (ISBI), pp. 870–873. IEEE, Beijing (2014). https://doi.org/10.1109/ISBI.2014.6868009

Improved Time-Resolved MRA Using k-Space Deep Learning

Eunju Cha[1], Eung Yeop Kim[2], and Jong Chul Ye[1]([✉])

[1] Korea Advanced Institute of Science and Technology,
Daejeon 34141, Republic of Korea
jong.ye@kaist.ac.kr

[2] Gachon University College of Medicine, Incheon 21565, Republic of Korea

Abstract. In dynamic contrast enhanced (DCE) MRI, temporal and spatial resolution can be improved by time-resolved angiography with interleaved stochastic trajectories (TWIST) thanks to its highly accelerated acquisitions. However, due to limited k-space samples, the periphery of the k-space data from several adjacent frames should be combined to reconstruct one temporal frame so that the temporal resolution of TWIST is limited. Furthermore, the k-space sampling patterns of TWIST imaging have been especially designed for a generalized autocalibrating partial parallel acquisition (GRAPPA) reconstruction. Therefore, the number of shared frames cannot be reduced to provide a reconstructed image with better temporal resolution. The purpose of this study is to improve the temporal resolution of TWIST using a novel k-space deep learning approach. Direct k-space interpolation is performed simultaneously for multiple coils by exploiting spatial domain redundancy and multi-coil diversity. Furthermore, the proposed method can provide the reconstructed images with various numbers of view sharing. Experimental results using in vivo TWIST data set showed the accuracy and the flexibility of the proposed method.

Keywords: Dynamic contrast enhanced MRI · Parallel imaging
Deep learning

1 Introduction

DCE-MRI is useful for the diagnosis of stroke or cancer because it provides information on the physiological characteristics of the tissue by imaging the flow of the contrast agent [16]. In particular, TWIST [11] imaging gives improved temporal and spatial resolution thanks to its highly accelerated acquisition. In TWIST, the high frequency regions of the k-space from multiple temporal frames should be combined to obtain uniformly sub-sampled k-space data so that GRAPPA [4] can be applied to reconstruct the data. However, the temporal resolution of

Supported by National Research Foundation of Korea, Grand number NRF2016R1A2B3008104.

F. Knoll et al. (Eds.): MLMIR 2018, LNCS 11074, pp. 47–54, 2018.
https://doi.org/10.1007/978-3-030-00129-2_6

TWIST is not a true one due to the view sharing of several temporal frames. In addition, since the k-space sampling patterns are designed for GRAPPA reconstruction, the number of view sharing is fixed after the data acquisition.

In our previous works [3], we proposed to improve temporal resolution of TWIST via k-space interpolation using ALOHA [8,12,14] which synergistically combines parallel MRI (pMRI) and CS-MRI. However, since the multiple matrix factorization is essential for applying ALOHA, the computational cost for the reconstruction of 4-dimensional TWIST imaging was too expensive. In addition, if the number of view sharing is not enough, the spatial resolution can be degraded. Therefore, new approach is required to overcome this limitation.

This paper aims at enhancing the temporal resolution of TWIST imaging by reducing the number of view sharing using deep learning. Furthermore, we proposed the algorithm that can generate reconstructed images at multiple number of view sharing to exploit the trade-off between spatial and temporal resolution. For our purposes, we need to deal with two major technical issues. First, unlike most of the deep learning approaches for MR reconstruction [6,10,13,15,17], our deep network needs to learn the k-space interpolation kernels for reconstruction at various number of view sharing. Second, with reduced view sharing, the reconstructed images using GRAPPA cannot be regarded as ground-truth data, so there is no label data for learning.

Based on the recent mathematical finding of the link between a deep convolutional neural network and a data-driven decomposition of Hankel matrix [18], here we propose a k-space deep network using the basic idea of ALOHA for parallel MRI [9], which is implemented in the k-space domain by stacking multi-coil k-space data along the channel direction of the network as shown in Fig. 1.

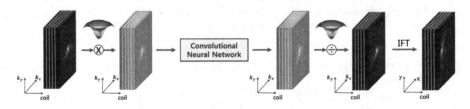

Fig. 1. An overall scheme of k-space deep learning for parallel MRI. IFT represents inverse Fourier transform.

Another major contribution of this paper is that our network learns the k-space interpolation relationship between the minimum number of k-space samples and completely sampled k-space data from GRAPPA reconstruction to address the lack of ground-truth data. As will be shown in later, this approach allows the trained network to provide accurate reconstruction results at various number of view sharing, since the network is trained to learn the Fourier domain features rather than image domain ones.

2   Theory

2.1   Problem Formulation

In TWIST, the center of k-space data (A region in Fig. 2) is more frequently sampled than the periphery of k-space data (B region in Fig. 2). Since it reduces the total number of samples for each frame, the reduced acquisition time is required. However, high frequency k-space data from several frames should be shared to make one time frame due to the strongly subsampled high frequency k-space data. Therefore, the actual temporal resolution of TWIST imaging is determined by the number of view-sharing.

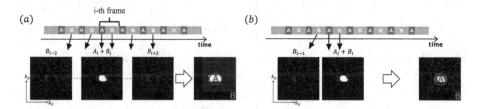

Fig. 2. The center and periphery of k-space are denoted by A and B, respectively. (a) Standard view sharing scheme for 2D GRAPPA reconstruction, and (b) an example of reduced view sharing scheme.

There are different types of view sharing. For example, as shown in Fig. 2(a), one type of view sharing is specifically designed for 2-D GRAPPA reconstruction, where high frequency regions of five time frames $(B_{i-2}, \cdots, B_{i+2})$ are combined to provide a 2-D uniform sub-sampled k-space data with downsampling factor of three and two along k_x and k_y directions, respectively.

Unlike the standard TWIST view sharing scheme, we are interested in using various number of reduced view sharing. For example, the number of view sharing can be reduced to two frames as shown in Fig. 2(b). GRAPPA cannot be applied to this irregular sampling pattern, so we proposed a multi-coil deep learning approach to reconstruct the k-space data.

2.2   From ALOHA to Deep Neural Network

ALOHA [9, 19] was developed based on the duality between the sparsity in image domain and the low-rankness of associated Hankel matrix in the k-space domain. In addition, for parallel MRI, there exists the k-space inter-coil annihilating filter relationship [9]:

$$\widehat{g}_i \circledast \widehat{s}_j - \widehat{g}_j \circledast \widehat{s}_i = 0, \quad \forall i \neq j, \tag{1}$$

where $\widehat{g}_i$ and $\widehat{s}_i$ denote k-space data of the i-th coil and the specturm of the i-th coil sensitivity map, respectively. This relationship in (1) leads to the low-rank property of the following extended Hankel structured matrix [9]:

$$\mathbb{H}_{d|P}(\widehat{\mathbf{G}}) = \left[\mathbb{H}_d(\widehat{\mathbf{g}}_1) \cdots \mathbb{H}_d(\widehat{\mathbf{g}}_P) \right] \tag{2}$$

where

$$\widehat{\mathbf{G}} = \left[\widehat{\mathbf{g}}_1 \cdots \widehat{\mathbf{g}}_P \right] \in \mathbb{C}^{N \times P}$$

with the k-space measurement $\widehat{\mathbf{g}}_i = \left[\widehat{g}_i(\mathbf{k}_1) \cdots \widehat{g}_i(\mathbf{k}_N) \right]^T$, and $\mathbb{H}_d(\widehat{\mathbf{g}}_i)$ is a Hankel matrix constructed from $\widehat{\mathbf{g}}_i$ with d denoting the matrix pencil size. P denotes the number of coils. Therefore, the missing elements of k-space data can be recovered using low rank Hankel matrix completion approaches [2,5]:

$$(MC) \quad \min_{\widehat{\mathbf{Z}} \in \mathbb{C}^{N \times P}} \quad \text{RANK } \mathbb{H}_{d|P}(\widehat{\mathbf{Z}}) \tag{3}$$

$$\text{subject to} \quad \mathcal{P}_\Lambda[\widehat{\mathbf{g}}_i] = \mathcal{P}_\Lambda[\widehat{\mathbf{z}}_i], \quad i = 1, \cdots, P,$$

where $\mathcal{P}_\Lambda$ is the downsampling operator $\mathcal{P}_\Lambda : \mathbb{C}^N \to \mathbb{C}^N$ defined as

$$[\mathcal{P}_\Lambda[\widehat{\mathbf{x}}]]_j = \begin{cases} [\widehat{\mathbf{x}}]_j & j \in \Lambda \\ 0, & \text{otherwise} \end{cases}. \tag{4}$$

However, this approach needs a relatively expensive computational cost for matrix factorization.

Recently, our group proposed k-space deep learning approaches for accelerated MRI [7] based on the observation that the Hankel matrix in the weighted k-space domain is low-ranked so that deep neural network can be efficiently implemented. By extending this idea, we apply the deep learning for the multi-channel k-space data by stacking the multi-coil k-space data along the channel direction of the network input.

3   Method

Four sets of in vivo 3D DCE data for carotid vessel imaging were acquired with a TWIST sequence using Siemens 3T Verio scanners. The scanning parameters for two sets were as following: repetition time (TR) $= 2.5$ ms, echo time (TE) $= 0.94$ ms, $159 \times 640 \times 80$ matrix, 2.5 mm slice thickness, 16 coils, and 37 temporal frames. For other two sets, the acquisition parameters were same as above, expect for 1.2 mm slice thickness and 30 temporal frames. The sampling pattern of data sets is illustrated in Fig. 2(a). Only 63% of data was acquired due to the partial Fourier. The downsampling factor was three and two along k_x and k_y direction, respectively. Among four patient data sets, three patient data sets were used for training and validation. We used the remaining one patient data set for test. The input k-space data for network is the k_x-k_y slice along z direction and temporal frames.

We employed the tight-frame U-net [18] thanks to its capability of preserving of the details of image. To deal with complex-valued multi-channel k-space

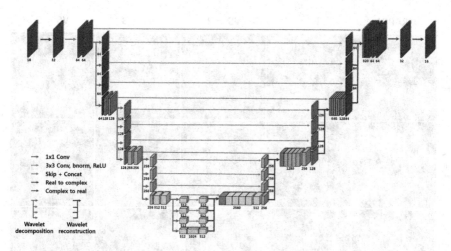

Fig. 3. Network architecture of tight-frame U-net.

data, we divide the complex-valued k-space data into real and imaginary channels similar to [7]. The interpolated k-space data can be formed from the real and imaginary channels as shown in Fig. 3. We implemented the network using TensorFlow library [1].

4 Result

Figure 4 showed the subtracted maximum intensity projection (MIP) images for test data. The temporal frames were selected to illustrate the propagation of the contrast agent. In the proposed method, we generated the reconstructed images using same neural network at various number of view sharing (VS). The raw data in Fig. 4 is obtained by directly apply inverse Fast Fourier Transform (FFT) to the k-space data without view sharing, which provide the true temporal resolution.

In the GRAPPA reconstruction, the contrast agent was suddenly propagated from the $T = 10$ frame to $T = 11$ frame as shown in Fig. 4. Since the degradation of temporal resolution can be caused by the combination of multiple temporal frames, the flow of contrast agent can be quickly changed only between one frame. In the reconstructed images with $VS = 2$ using the proposed method, the dynamics of the contrast agent is correctly demonstrated. As shown in Fig. 4, the degree of temporal blurring in $T = 11$ frame can be captured depending on the number of view sharing. The results of proposed method with $VS = 5$, which is same to the conventional method, provided very similar spatial and temporal resolution to the GRAPPA reconstruction.

Furthermore, the computational cost of the proposed method is more efficient than that of GRAPPA and ALOHA. The proposed method can produce the result only in 0.029 s, which is several order of magnitude faster than GRAPPA and ALOHA.

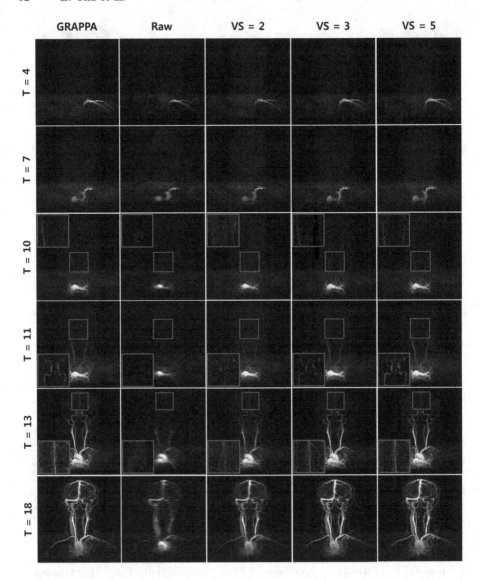

Fig. 4. Subtracted MIP results of GRPPA, raw data and the proposed methods for various number of view sharing. VS stands for the number of view sharing.

5   Conclusion

In this paper, to enhance the temporal resolution of TWIST imaging and to develop an algorithm that generates reconstruction results at various sliding window size, we proposed a novel k-space deep learning algorithm for parallel MRI. Our k-space deep network can exploit the redundancies along the coil and image domain. The experimental results showed that one trained network can provide multiple reconstruction results with various spatial and temporal resolution by changing the number of view sharing for the network input. We believe that the proposed method suggests a significant new research direction that can extend the clinical applications.

References

1. Abadi, M., et al.: TensorFlow: a system for large-scale machine learning. In: OSDI, vol. 16, pp. 265–283 (2016)
2. Candès, E.J., Recht, B.: Exact matrix completion via convex optimization. Found. Comput. Math. **9**(6), 717–772 (2009)
3. Cha, E., Jin, K.H., Kim, E.Y., Ye, J.C.: True temporal resolution TWIST imaging using annihilating filter-based low-rank wrap around Hankel matrix. In: The International Society for Magnetic Resonance in Medicine. ISMRM (2017)
4. Griswold, M.A., et al.: Generalized autocalibrating partially parallel acquisitions (GRAPPA). Magn. Reson. Med. **47**(6), 1202–1210 (2002)
5. Gross, D.: Recovering low-rank matrices from few coefficients in any basis. IEEE Trans. Inf. Theory **57**(3), 1548–1566 (2011)
6. Han, Y.S., Yoo, J., Ye, J.C.: Deep learning with domain adaptation for accelerated projection reconstruction. In: MR. Magnetic Resonance in Medicine (2018). https://doi.org/10.1002/mrm.27106
7. Han, Y., Ye, J.C.: k-Space Deep Learning for Accelerated MRI. arXiv preprint arXiv:1805.03779 (2018)
8. Jin, K., Lee, D., Ye, J.: A general framework for compressed sensing and parallel MRI using annihilating filter based low-rank Hankel matrix. IEEE Trans. Comput. Imaging **PP**(99), 1 (2016). https://doi.org/10.1109/TCI.2016.2601296
9. Jin, K.H., Lee, D., Ye, J.C.: A general framework for compressed sensing and parallel MRI using annihilating filter based low-rank Hankel matrix. IEEE Trans. Comput. Imaging **2**(4), 480–495 (2016)
10. Kwon, K., Kim, D., Park, H.: A parallel MR imaging method using multilayer perceptron. Med. Phys. **44**(12), 6209–6224 (2017)
11. Laub, G., Kroeker, R.: syngo TWIST for dynamic time-resolved MR angiography. Magnetom Flash **34**(3), 92–95 (2006)
12. Lee, D., Jin, K.H., Kim, E.Y., Park, S.H., Ye, J.C.: Acceleration of MR parameter mapping using annihilating filter-based low rank Hankel matrix (ALOHA). Magnetic Reson. Med. **76**(6), 1848–1864 (2016)
13. Lee, D., Yoo, J., Tak, S., Ye, J.: Deep residual learning for accelerated MRI using magnitude and phase networks. IEEE Trans. Biomed. Eng. (2018)
14. Lee, J., Jin, K.H., Ye, J.C.: Reference-free single-pass EPI Nyquist ghost correction using annihilating filter-based low rank Hankel matrix (ALOHA). Magnetic Reson. Med. **76**(6), 1775–1789 (2016)
15. Quan, T.M., Nguyen-Duc, T., Jeong, W.K.: Compressed sensing MRI reconstruction using a generative adversarial network with a cyclic loss. IEEE Trans. Med. Imaging (2018, in press)
16. Turnbull, L.W.: Dynamic contrast-enhanced MRI in the diagnosis and management of breast cancer. NMR Biomed. **22**(1), 28–39 (2009)

17. Wang, S., et al.: Accelerating magnetic resonance imaging via deep learning. In: 2016 IEEE 13th International Symposium on Biomedical Imaging (ISBI), pp. 514–517. IEEE (2016)
18. Ye, J.C., Han, Y., Cha, E.: Deep convolutional framelets: a general deep learning framework for inverse problems. SIAM J. Imaging Sci. **11**(2), 991–1048 (2018)
19. Ye, J.C., Kim, J.M., Jin, K.H., Lee, K.: Compressive sampling using annihilating filter-based low-rank interpolation. IEEE Trans. Inf. Theory **63**(2), 777–801 (2017)

Joint Motion Estimation and Segmentation from Undersampled Cardiac MR Image

Chen Qin[1]([✉]), Wenjia Bai[1], Jo Schlemper[1], Steffen E. Petersen[2],
Stefan K. Piechnik[3], Stefan Neubauer[3], and Daniel Rueckert[1]

[1] Department of Computing, Imperial College London, London, UK
c.qin15@imperial.ac.uk
[2] NIHR Biomedical Research Centre at Barts, Queen Mary University of London,
London, UK
[3] Division of Cardiovascular Medicine, Radcliffe Department of Medicine,
University of Oxford, Oxford, UK

Abstract. Accelerating the acquisition of magnetic resonance imaging
(MRI) is a challenging problem, and many works have been proposed
to reconstruct images from undersampled k-space data. However, if the
main purpose is to extract certain quantitative measures from the images,
perfect reconstructions may not always be necessary as long as the images
enable the means of extracting the clinically relevant measures. In this
paper, we work on jointly predicting cardiac motion estimation and segmentation directly from undersampled data, which are two important
steps in quantitatively assessing cardiac function and diagnosing cardiovascular diseases. In particular, a unified model consisting of both motion
estimation branch and segmentation branch is learned by optimising the
two tasks simultaneously. Additional corresponding fully-sampled images
are incorporated into the network as a parallel sub-network to enhance
and guide the learning during the training process. Experimental results
using cardiac MR images from 220 subjects show that the proposed
model is robust to undersampled data and is capable of predicting results
that are close to that from fully-sampled ones, while bypassing the usual
image reconstruction stage.

1 Introduction

Cardiac magnetic resonance imaging (MRI) provides qualitative and quantitative information of the morphology and function of the heart, which are crucial
for assessing cardiovascular diseases. Both cardiac MR image segmentation and
motion estimation are essential steps for the dynamic exploration of the cardiac
function. However, one limitation of the cardiovascular MR is the low acquisition speed due to both hardware and physiological constraints. Most approaches
consider undersampling the data in k-space and then reconstruct the images
[7,9]. Nevertheless, in most cases, perfect reconstructions are not necessary as

© Springer Nature Switzerland AG 2018
F. Knoll et al. (Eds.): MLMIR 2018, LNCS 11074, pp. 55–63, 2018.
https://doi.org/10.1007/978-3-030-00129-2_7

long as the images allow to obtain accurate clinically relevant parameters such as changes in ventricular volumes and the elasticity and contractility properties of the myocardium. Therefore, instead of firstly recovering non-aliased images, it may be more effective to estimate the final results directly from undersampled MR data and also to make such estimations as accurate as possible.

In this paper, we propose to learn a joint deep learning network for cardiac motion estimation and segmentation directly from undersampled cardiac MR data, bypassing the MR reconstruction process. In particular, we extend the joint model proposed in [6] which consists of an unsupervised cardiac motion estimation branch and a weakly-supervised segmentation branch, where the two tasks share the same feature encoder. We investigate the network's capability of predicting motion estimation and segmentation maps simultaneously and directly from undersampled cardiac MR data. The problem is formulated by incorporating supervision from fully sampled MR image pairs in addition to the composite loss function as proposed in [6]. Simulation experiments have been performed on 220 subjects under different acceleration factors with radial undersampling patterns. Experiments indicate that results learned directly from undersampled data are reasonably accurate and are close to predictions from fully-sampled data. This could potentially lead to future works that enable fast and accurate analysis in an integrated MRI reconstruction and analysis pipeline.

1.1 Related Work

Cardiac segmentation and motion estimation are well studied problems in medical imaging. Traditionally, most approaches consider these two tasks separately [1,11,12]. However, it is known that segmentation and motion estimation problems are closely related, and optimising these two tasks jointly has been proven to improve the performance for both challenges. Recently, Oksuz et al. [5] proposed a joint optimisation scheme for registration and segmentation using dictionary learning based descriptors, which enables better performance for both of these ill-posed processes. Qin et al. [6] proposed a unified deep learning model for both cardiac motion estimation and segmentation, where no motion ground truth is required and only temporally sparse annotated frames in a cardiac cycle are needed.

However, there are only a limited number of works that focus on obtaining segmentation maps and motion fields directly from undersampled MR data. One direction of the research is on the application-driven MRI [2], where an integrated acquisition-reconstruction-segmentation process was adopted to provide a more efficient and accurate solution. Schlemper et al. [10] expanded on the idea of application-driven MRI and presented an end-to-end synthesis network and a latent feature interpolation network to predict segmentation maps from extremely undersampled dynamic MR data. Our work focuses on the scenario where motion fields and segmentation maps can be jointly predicted directly from undersampled MR data, bypassing the usual MR image reconstruction stage.

2 Methods

Our goal is to predict the simultaneous motion estimation and segmentation directly from undersampled cardiac MR images and make sure that such predictions are as accurate and efficient as possible. Here we extend the effective unified model (Motion-Seg Net) proposed in [6] to adapt to the application for undersampled MR data. The proposed network architecture consists of two branches which perform motion estimation and segmentation jointly, and a well-trained sub-network for fully-sampled images is incorporated to provide additional supervision during the training process. Note that at test stage, only the undersampled sub-network is needed, and no fully-sampled data is required. The overall architecture of the model is shown in Fig. 1.

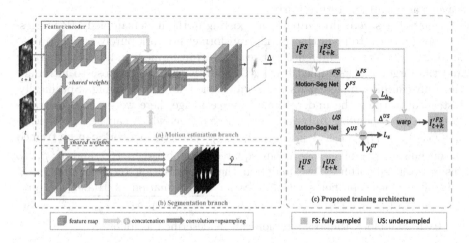

Fig. 1. The overall schematic architecture of proposed network for joint estimation of cardiac motion and segmentation directly from undersampled data. (a) (b) The Motion-Seg net adopted from [6]. (c) Proposed architecture for training the Motion-Seg net on undersampled data. US: undersampled, FS: fully-sampled

2.1 Unsupervised Cardiac Motion Estimation from Undersampled MR Image

Inspired by the success of the joint prediction network proposed in [6] which effectively learns useful representations, here we propose to adapt the network to undersampled MR data. In contrast to the fully-sampled case where only self-supervision is required for the motion estimation, it is difficult for the undersampled images to merely rely on self-supervision, i.e., the intensity difference, due to the noises caused by aliased patterns. To address this, we propose to incorporate their corresponding fully-sampled image pairs as an additional supervision to guide the training for the undersampled images, and a schematic illustration of the model is shown in Fig. 1(a) and (c).

The task is to find an optical flow representation between the target undersampled frame I_t^{US} and the source undersampled frame I_{t+k}^{US}, where the output is a pixel-wise 2D motion field Δ^{US} representing the displacement in x and y directions. We exploit a modified version of the network proposed in [6] for the representation learning, in which it mainly consists of three components: a Siamese network for the feature extraction of both target frame and source frame where the encoder is adapted from VGG-16 Net; a multi-scale concatenation of features from pairs of frames motivated by the traditional multi-level registration method [8]; and a bilinear interpolation sampler that warps the source frame to the target one by using the estimated displacement field $\Delta^{US} = (\Delta^{US}x, \Delta^{US}y; \theta_\Delta^{US})$, where the network is parameterised by θ_Δ^{US} which is learned directly from undersampled MR data. Note that a RNN unit could be potentially incorporated to propagate motion information along the temporal dimension [6], and we will leave it as one of our future work.

Due to the severe aliased patterns existing in the undersampled MR images, it is not practical to train the spatial transformer network purely based on minimising the intensity difference between the transformed undersampled frame and the target undersampled frame. To address this, we propose to introduce the fully-sampled image pairs as a supervision for the training. Specifically, instead of warping the undersampled source image, here we propose to transform the corresponding fully-sampled source image, which can be expressed as $I_{t+k}^{'FS}(x,y) = \Gamma\{I_{t+k}^{FS}(x + \Delta_{t+k}^{US}x, y + \Delta_{t+k}^{US}y)\}$. Then the network can be trained by optimising the pixel-wise mean squared error between I_t^{FS} and $I_{t+k}^{'FS}$. To ensure local smoothness, we maintain the regularisation term for the gradients of displacement fields which uses an approximation of Huber loss proposed in [3,6], namely $\mathcal{H}(\delta_{x,y}\Delta^{US}) = \sqrt{\epsilon + \sum_{i=x,y}(\delta_x\Delta^{US}i^2 + \delta_y\Delta^{US}i^2)}$, where $\epsilon = 0.01$. Therefore, the loss function can be described as follows:

$$\mathcal{L}_m = \frac{1}{N_s} \sum_{(I_t, I_{t+k}) \in S} [\|I_t^{FS} - I_{t+k}^{'FS}\|^2 + \alpha\mathcal{H}(\delta_{x,y}\Delta_{t+k}^{US})], \tag{1}$$

where N_s stands for the number of sample pairs in the training set S, and α is a regularisation parameter to trade off between image dissimilarity and local smoothness.

However, it is observed that for heavily undersampled images, such weak supervision in Eq. 1 is not sufficient. Therefore, in order to push the learning results from undersampled data to be as accurate as that from fully-sampled data, we additionally introduce a pixel-wise mean squared error loss on the displacement fields between the estimation from undersampled data (Δ_{t+k}^{US}) and that from fully-sampled one (Δ_{t+k}^{FS}). Since only the motion of anatomical structures is of interest, here we propose to mask the region of interests (ROI) by utilising the predicted segmentation maps from fully-sampled data to allow that only errors from ROI can be backpropagated to contribute to the learning. The proposed loss term can be expressed as $\mathcal{L}_{\Delta_{t+k}} = \|(\Delta_{t+k}^{US} - \Delta_{t+k}^{FS}) * \mathbf{M}_t\|^2$, where $\mathbf{M}_t$ is a one-hot mask (1 for ROI, and 0 for background) generated from the segmentation maps from frame t of fully-sampled images. Thus, the overall loss function for motion estimation is as follows:

$$\mathcal{L}_m = \frac{1}{N_s} \sum \left[\|I_t^{FS} - I_{t+k}'^{FS}\|^2 + \alpha \mathcal{H}(\delta_{x,y}\Delta_{t+k}^{US}) + \beta \|(\Delta_{t+k}^{US} - \Delta_{t+k}^{FS}) * \mathbf{M}_t\|^2 \right], \quad (2)$$

in which an additional trade-off parameter β is introduced. Note that no ground truth displacement fields are required during the training, thus the motion is still estimated unsupervisedly.

2.2 Joint Cardiac Motion Estimation and Segmentation from Undersampled MR Image

Previous works have shown that motion estimation and segmentation tasks are complementary [4,6,13]. Therefore, here we couples both tasks for the joint prediction from undersampled MR data. The schematic architecture of the unified model is shown in Fig. 1.

The joint model consists of two branches: the motion estimation branch proposed in Sect. 2.1 which introduces additional supervision from fully sampled images, and the segmentation branch based on the network proposed in [1], where both branches share the joint feature encoder (Siamese style network) as shown in Fig. 1. As images are only temporally sparse annotated, predictions from corresponding fully-sampled images are used as supervision for those unlabelled data. Therefore a categorical cross-entropy loss $\mathcal{L}_s = -\sum_{l \in L} y_l^{GT} \log(f(x_l; \Theta^{US})) - \sum_{n \in U} \hat{y}_n^{FS} \log(f(x_n; \Theta^{US}))$ on labelled data set L and unlabelled data set U is used for segmentation branch, in which we define x_l and x_n as the input data, y_l^{GT} as the ground truth, $\hat{y}_n^{FS}$ is predictions from fully-sampled images and f is the segmentation function parameterised by Θ^{US}. Different from the loss function as stated in [6], here we don't employ the loss $\mathcal{L}_w$ between the warped segmentations and the target, as we find that for undersampled cases, minimising $\mathcal{L}_w$ could introduce more noises and uncertainties into the network training presumably because of the less accurate predictions. We empirically observed that this could lead to a small performance degradation especially for the segmentation branch.

As a result, the overall loss function for the joint model can be defined as:

$$\mathcal{L} = \mathcal{L}_m + \lambda \mathcal{L}_s, \quad (3)$$

where λ is a trade-off parameter for balancing these two tasks. $\mathcal{L}_m$ can be of the form of Eq. 1 or Eq. 2, and we will examine their comparisons in experiments.

3 Experiments and Results

Experiments were performed on 220 short-axis cardiac MR sequences from UK Biobank study. Each scan contains a sequence of 50 frames, where manual segmentations of left-ventricular (LV) cavity, the myocardium (Myo) and the right-ventricular (RV) cavity are available on ED and ES frames. A short-axis image stack typically consists of 10 image slices, and the pixel resolution is $1.8 \times 1.8 \times 10.0 \ mm^3$. Since only magnitude images are available, here we employed a phase map synthesis scheme proposed in [10] to synthetically generate phase maps (smoothly varying 2D sinusoid waves), in order to convert magnitude images to complex valued images and to make the simulation more realistic. In experiments, the synthesised complex valued images were back-transformed to regenerate k-space samples. The input undersampled images were generated by randomly undersampling the k-space samples using uniform radial undersampling patterns. For pre-processing, all training images were cropped to the same size of 192×192, and intensity was normalized to the range of [0,1]. In our experiments, we split the data into 100/100/20 for training/testing/validation. Parameters used in the loss function were set to be $\alpha = 0.001$, $\beta = 1$, and $\lambda = 0.01$, which were chosen via validation set. Fully-sampled sub-network parameters were loaded from [6], and we train the undersampled network using Adam optimiser with a learning rate of 0.0001. Data augmentation was performed on-the-fly, with random rotation, translation, and scaling.

As work [6] has already shown that the joint model can significantly outperform model with single branch, in this work, we mainly focus on the evaluation of the performance on undersampled data. We first evaluated the performance of motion estimation by comparing the proposed model with a B-spline free-form deformation (FFD) algorithm[1] [8], and the results are shown in Table 1. Here we examined the effect of different losses on the model's performance, where we termed method using $\mathcal{L}_m$ with the form of Eq. 1 as Proposed-A, and the one using Eq. 2 as Proposed-B. Motion fields were estimated between ES and ED frame, and mean contour distance (MCD) and Hausdorff distance (HD) were computed between the warped ES segmentations and ED segmentations. Results on fully-sampled (FS) images are presented in Table 1 as a reference. It can be observed that proposed methods consistently outperform FFD on all acceleration rates with $p \ll 0.001$ using Wilcoxon signed rank test, and is able to produce results that are close to the fully-sampled images. Furthermore, it can also be noticed that for higher acceleration rates ($6\times$ and $8\times$), Proposed-B produces significantly better results than Proposed-A ($p \ll 0.001$). This is reflected by the fact that higher undersampling rates result in more aliased images, therefore a relatively strong supervision ($\mathcal{L}_\Delta$) is more needed to guide the learning in comparison to images with less aliasing ($3\times$).

We further evaluated the segmentation performance of the model on undersampled data with different acceleration factors. Results reported in Table 2 are Dice scores computed with manual annotations on LV, Myo, and RV, as well as the clinical parameter ejection fraction (EF). It has been observed that Proposed-A and Proposed-B didn't differ significantly in terms of segmentation performance, so here we only report results obtained from Proposed-B in Table 2. It can be seen that though there is a relatively small drop of performance as acceleration factors increase, the network is robust to train on undersampled

---

[1] https://github.com/BioMedIA/MIRTK.

Table 1. Evaluation of motion estimation accuracy for undersampled MR data with different acceleration factors in terms of the mean contour distance (MCD) and Hausdorff distance (HD) in mm (mean and standard deviation). Loss function using $\mathcal{L}_m$(Eq. 1) is termed as Proposed-A, and the one using $\mathcal{L}_m$(Eq. 2) is termed as Proposed-B. Bold numbers indicate the best results for different undersampling rates.

Method		MCD			HD		
		LV	Myo	RV	LV	Myo	RV
FS	FFD	1.83 (0.53)	2.47 (0.74)	3.53 (1.25)	5.10 (1.28)	6.47 (1.69)	12.04 (4.85)
	Joint model [6]	**1.30 (0.34)**	**1.19 (0.26)**	**3.03 (1.08)**	**3.52 (0.82)**	**3.43 (0.87)**	**11.38 (4.34)**
3×	FFD	2.19 (0.49)	2.54 (0.74)	3.94 (1.38)	6.27 (1.64)	6.62 (1.72)	13.92 (5.03)
	Proposed-A	**1.32 (0.40)**	**1.23 (0.31)**	**3.41 (1.22)**	**3.53 (0.89)**	3.59 (1.10)	**12.69 (4.47)**
	Proposed-B	1.37 (0.45)	**1.23 (0.31)**	3.44 (1.22)	3.59 (0.98)	**3.55 (1.10)**	**12.69 (4.45)**
6×	FFD	2.80 (0.77)	2.74 (0.75)	4.48 (1.46)	7.83 (2.30)	7.26 (2.26)	15.63 (5.19)
	Proposed-A	2.10 (0.80)	1.44 (0.38)	3.84 (1.27)	4.79 (1.40)	3.98 (1.26)	13.45 (4.49)
	Proposed-B	**1.74 (0.68)**	**1.34 (0.35)**	**3.68 (1.27)**	**4.20 (1.30)**	**3.77 (1.21)**	**13.08 (4.49)**
8×	FFD	3.29 (0.97)	3.09 (0.99)	4.94 (1.67)	9.40 (2.70)	8.48 (3.05)	17.16 (5.75)
	Proposed-A	2.30 (0.97)	1.52 (0.46)	4.02 (1.37)	5.19 (1.71)	4.16 (1.32)	13.79 (4.60)
	Proposed-B	**1.79 (0.70)**	**1.44 (0.39)**	**3.76 (1.30)**	**4.36 (1.40)**	**3.97 (1.28)**	**13.27 (4.55)**

data, and the clinical parameter predicted directly from undersampled data is very close to that from fully-sampled images. Furthermore, a visualisation result of the network predictions on 8× accelerated data in a cardiac cycle is shown in Fig. 2, where myocardial motion indicated by the yellow arrows were established between ED and other time frames. Overall, predictions directly from undersampled MR data are reasonably accurate, despite some small underestimations.

Table 2. Evaluation of segmentation performance under different acceleration factors in terms of Dice Metric (mean and standard deviation) and average percentage (%) error for ejection fraction (EF) compared with fully-sampled data.

Acceleration	LV	Myo	RV	EF
FS [6]	**0.9348 (0.0408)**	**0.8640 (0.0295)**	0.8861 (0.0453)	-
3×	0.9303 (0.0450)	0.8596 (0.0309)	**0.8884 (0.0433)**	2.68%
6×	0.9214 (0.0475)	0.8424 (0.0310)	0.8804 (0.0456)	3.56%
8×	0.9141 (0.0487)	0.8260 (0.0343)	0.8658 (0.0523)	4.16%

4   Conclusion

In this paper, we explored the joint motion estimation and segmentation directly from undersampled cardiac MR data, bypassing the usual image reconstruction stage. The proposed method takes advantage of a unified model which shares the same feature encoder for both tasks and performs them simultaneously. In particular, we additionally introduced a parallel well-trained sub-network for

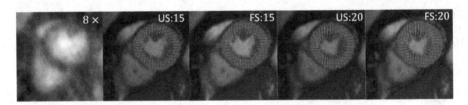

Fig. 2. Comparison visualisation results for simultaneous prediction of motion estimation and segmentation on data with undersampling rates 8. Myocardial motions are from ED to other time points (numbers on the top right). Segmentations are overlaid on fully-sampled data for better visualisation.

corresponding fully-sampled MR image pairs as a supervision source for training undersampled data, in order to push the predictions from undersampled data to be as accurate as possible. We showed that the proposed network is robust to undersampled data, and results predicted directly from undersampled images are close to that from fully-sampled ones, which could potentially enable fast analysis for MR imaging. In the future, it is also interesting to explore methods that are independent of aliased patterns and acceleration factors.

References

1. Bai, W., Sinclair, M., Tarroni, G., et al.: Automated cardiovascular magnetic resonance image analysis with fully convolutional networks. J. Cardiovasc. Magn. Reson. (2018)
2. Caballero, J., Bai, W., Price, A.N., Rueckert, D., Hajnal, J.V.: Application-driven MRI: joint reconstruction and segmentation from undersampled MRI data. In: Golland, P., Hata, N., Barillot, C., Hornegger, J., Howe, R. (eds.) MICCAI 2014. LNCS, vol. 8673, pp. 106–113. Springer, Cham (2014). https://doi.org/10.1007/978-3-319-10404-1_14
3. Caballero, J., Ledig, C., Aitken, A., et al.: Real-time video super-resolution with spatio-temporal networks and motion compensation. In: CVPR (2017)
4. Cheng, J., Tsai, Y.H., Wang, S., Yang, M.H.: SegFlow: Joint learning for video object segmentation and optical flow. In: ICCV, pp. 686–695 (2017)
5. Oksuz, I., Dharmakumar, R., Tsaftaris, S.A.: Joint myocardial registration and segmentation of cardiac BOLD MRI. In: Pop, M., Sermesant, M., Jodoin, P.-M., Lalande, A., Zhuang, X., Yang, G., Young, A., Bernard, O. (eds.) STACOM 2017. LNCS, vol. 10663, pp. 12–20. Springer, Cham (2018). https://doi.org/10.1007/978-3-319-75541-0_2
6. Qin, C., et al.: Joint learning of motion estimation and segmentation for cardiac MR image sequences. arXiv preprint arXiv:1806.04066 (2018)
7. Qin, C., Schlemper, J., Caballero, J., Price, A., Hajnal, J.V., Rueckert, D.: Convolutional recurrent neural networks for dynamic MR image reconstruction. arXiv preprint arXiv:1712.01751 (2017)
8. Rueckert, D., Sonoda, L.I., Hayes, C.: Nonrigid registration using free-form deformations: application to breast MR images. IEEE Trans. Med. Imaging **18**(8), 712–721 (1999)

9. Schlemper, J., Caballero, J., Hajnal, J.V., Price, A., Rueckert, D.: A deep cascade of convolutional neural networks for dynamic MR image reconstruction. IEEE Trans. Med. Imaging **37**(2), 491–503 (2018)

10. Schlemper, J., Oktay, O., Bai, W., et al.: Cardiac MR segmentation from undersampled k-space using deep latent representation learning. In: MICCAI (2018)

11. Shi, W., Zhuang, X., Wang, H.: A comprehensive cardiac motion estimation framework using both untagged and 3-D tagged MR images based on nonrigid registration. IEEE Trans. Med. Imaging **31**(6), 1263–1275 (2012)

12. Tobon-Gomez, C., De Craene, M., Mcleod, K.: Benchmarking framework for myocardial tracking and deformation algorithms: an open access database. Med. Image Anal. **17**(6), 632–648 (2013)

13. Tsai, Y.H., Yang, M.H., Black, M.J.: Video segmentation via object flow. In: CVPR, pp. 3899–3908 (2016)

Bayesian Deep Learning for Accelerated MR Image Reconstruction

Jo Schlemper[1](✉), Daniel C. Castro[1], Wenjia Bai[1], Chen Qin[1], Ozan Oktay[1],
Jinming Duan[1], Anthony N. Price[2], Jo Hajnal[2], and Daniel Rueckert[1]

[1] Biomedical Image Analysis Group, Imperial College London, London, UK
{js3611,dc315,w.bai,c.qin15,o.oktay13,j.duan,d.rueckert}@imperial.ac.uk
[2] Imaging and Biomedical Engineering Clinical Academic Group,
King's College London, London, UK
{anthony.price,jo.hajnal}@kcl.ac.uk

Abstract. Recently, many deep learning (DL) based MR image reconstruction methods have been proposed with promising results. However, only a handful of work has been focussing on *characterising* the behaviour of deep networks, such as investigating when the networks may fail to reconstruct. In this work, we explore the applicability of Bayesian DL techniques to model the uncertainty associated with DL-based reconstructions. In particular, we apply MC-dropout and heteroscedastic loss to the reconstruction networks to model *epistemic* and *aleatoric* uncertainty. We show that the proposed Bayesian methods achieve competitive performance when the test images are relatively far from the training data distribution and outperforms when the baseline method is overparametrised. In addition, we qualitatively show that there seems to be a correlation between the magnitude of the produced uncertainty maps and the error maps, demonstrating the potential utility of the Bayesian DL methods for assessing the reliability of the reconstructed images.

1 Introduction

Deep learning (DL)-based accelerated magnetic resonance (MR) image reconstruction is currently an active area of research. Many model architectures have been proposed, such as networks which learn end-to-end transformations [4], networks which "unroll" the traditional optimisation algorithm into a deep network [7,9], optimisation algorithms incorporating deep priors [11] and, more recently, networks incorporating adversarial losses [12]. Finding the optimal network architecture remains an exciting problem. Despite there being an advance in architectural search, only marginal progress has been made in understanding the reconstruction networks' behaviour. In [13], the expressibility of the network to achieve a perfect reconstruction is outlined using the connection between convolutional neural networks (CNN) and convolution framelets. The authors of [6] empirically assessed the generalisability of the variational inference network, and found that the performance of the network is sensitive to the signal-to-noise ratio (SNR) of data. Nevertheless, no theory exists which can explain the worst-case

© Springer Nature Switzerland AG 2018
F. Knoll et al. (Eds.): MLMIR 2018, LNCS 11074, pp. 64–71, 2018.
https://doi.org/10.1007/978-3-030-00129-2_8

behaviour of these networks. In [1], it is shown that methods with adversarial losses can bias the reconstruction with the risk of hallucination. Even though DL methods are shown effective, having a good grasp of how they produce error is crucial for the reliable deployment of these methods in clinical settings.

While bridging the gap in our theoretical understanding of DL-based reconstruction remains challenging, the literature from *Bayesian deep learning* suggests that the uncertainty associated with network outputs can be directly modelled using practical regularisation techniques [2]. Namely, these techniques are MC-dropout and heteroscedastic loss [5], which capture *model* uncertainty and *data* uncertainty respectively. Although such techniques have been applied to MR image quality transfer/super-resolution (SR) tasks [10], it is yet to be investigated for the general MR image reconstruction setting. In this work, we apply them to two network architectures, UNET [4] and a deep cascade of CNNs (DC-CNN) [9]. We show that the Bayesian DL methods are able to approximately characterise the confidence associated with the generated reconstructions. However, we also point out that the proposed formulation seems to be overly simplistic to model the "true" uncertainty associated with MR reconstruction problem in general. More sophisticated approaches may be necessary before such uncertainty maps can be leveraged in practical scenarios.

2   Methods

Problem Formulation: Let $\mathbf{x} \in \mathbb{C}^n$ be a fully-sampled image, $\mathbf{y} \in \mathbb{C}^m$ be the undersampled data obtained as $\mathbf{y} = \mathcal{F}_u \mathbf{x} + \epsilon$, where $\mathcal{F}_u$ is an undersampling Fourier operator and $\epsilon \sim \mathcal{N}(0, \sigma^2 \mathbf{I})$. The goal is to learn the inversion $p(\mathbf{x}|\mathbf{y})$ or $p(\mathbf{x}|\mathbf{x}_u)$ where $\mathbf{x}_u = \mathcal{F}_u^H \mathbf{y}$ is the zero-filled reconstruction, which is aliased. This is typically approached by a maximum *a posteriori* (MAP) estimate $\arg\max_{\mathbf{x}} p(\mathbf{x}|\mathbf{y}) = \arg\min_{\mathbf{x}} -\log p(\mathbf{y}|\mathbf{x}) - \log p(\mathbf{x})$ because this can be equivalently solved as a minimisation problem, wherein the likelihood and the prior terms correspond to data fidelity and regularisation terms, respectively. For example, compressed sensing can be seen as a MAP inference with sparsity-inducing prior. Many deep learning algorithms can be seen as an *approximation* to such MAP inference [3,7,9], where they learn an inversion function $f^{\mathbf{w}}(\mathbf{x}_u) \approx \mathbf{x}$, and the network parameters $\mathbf{w}$ are learnt from the dataset $\mathcal{D} = (\mathbf{Y}, \mathbf{X}) = (\{\mathbf{y}_1, \dots, \mathbf{y}_n\}, \{\mathbf{x}_1, \dots, \mathbf{x}_n\})$. The problem with MAP inference is that it provides only a point estimate. In the case of compressed sensing, there is a theoretical framework that relates the number of measurements, sparsity level and reconstruction error. For deep learning, no such theoretical properties exist yet and it is unknown when the network *fails* to reconstruct an image. Therefore, it is desirable to model the distribution $p(\mathbf{x}|\mathbf{y})$ instead, which can provide the variance associated with the output.

Bayesian Deep Learning: In the Bayesian formulation, given a new undersampled image $\mathbf{x}_u$ and dataset $\mathcal{D}$, a predictive distribution for the reconstructed image $\mathbf{x}$ is obtained by $p(\mathbf{x}|\mathbf{x}_u, \mathcal{D}) = \int p(\mathbf{x}|\mathbf{x}_u, \mathbf{w}) p(\mathbf{w}|\mathcal{D}) \, d\mathbf{w}$. Note that in practice the posterior $p(\mathbf{w}|\mathcal{D})$ is intractable and often approximated using a distribution $q(\mathbf{w})$ (*variational inference*). In addition, the above predictive distribution is often estimated via Monte Carlo integration unless an analytical solution exists.

There are two types of uncertainty that can be identified in general. The first kind is called *aleatoric* (data) uncertainty: this is irreducible uncertainty observed in data. For MR image reconstruction problem, besides measurement noise, there is an inherently high level of ambiguity whether a pixel value represents an aliasing pattern, some anatomy or a texture. Whenever the network encounters unseen pathological examples, the model should exhibit higher level of uncertainty for such region in the reconstruction. The second kind is called *epistemic* (model) uncertainty: given dataset $\mathcal{D}$, there are many plausible network parameters $\mathbf{w}$ that can reconstruct the data well. This can be reduced by increasing the size of $\mathcal{D}$, however, in medical imaging domain, it is often difficult to collect large training data and hence it is increasingly important to account for the variability in network output caused by this uncertainty.

The two types of uncertainty can be modelled by incorporating *heteroscedastic loss* and *MC-dropout* respectively. Here we only summarise the method, however, the detailed derivation can be found in [2,5]. Firstly, we set our likelihood function to be given by $p(\mathbf{x}|\mathbf{x}_u, \mathbf{w}) = \mathcal{N}(\mathbf{x}|f^{\mathbf{w}}(\mathbf{x}_u), g^{\mathbf{w}}(\mathbf{x}_u))$, where $f^{\mathbf{w}}(\mathbf{x}_u)$ models the mean prediction and $g^{\mathbf{w}}(\mathbf{x}_u)$ accounts for the uncertainty found in the input to estimate the covariance in the prediction. For simplicity, the covariance matrix is assumed to be diagonal (i.e. we only model the pixel-wise variance). The two networks are trained by minimising the heteroscedastic loss:

$$\mathcal{L}_{\text{Het.}}(\mathbf{w}) = \frac{1}{N|\mathcal{D}|} \sum_{(\mathbf{x}_u,\mathbf{x})\in\mathcal{D}} \sum_{i=1}^{N} \frac{1}{2g_i^{\mathbf{w}}(\mathbf{x}_u)} \|\mathbf{x}_i - f_i^{\mathbf{w}}(\mathbf{x}_u)\|^2 + \frac{1}{2} \log g_i^{\mathbf{w}}(\mathbf{x}_u), \quad (1)$$

i.e. the pixel-wise error is weighted by the predicted inverse pixel variance. Epistemic uncertainty can be modelled using *MC-dropout*: it simply applies dropout to the network activation maps. At test time, the predictive mean is given by $\mathbb{E}[\mathbf{x}] \approx \frac{1}{T}\sum_{t=1}^{T} f^{\mathbf{w}_t}(\mathbf{x}_u)$, where $\mathbf{w}_t$ denotes the network configuration after dropout has been applied. The predictive variance is given by $\mathbb{V}[\mathbf{x}] \approx \frac{1}{T}\sum_{t=1}^{T} g^{\mathbf{w}_t}(\mathbf{x}_u) + \frac{1}{T}\sum_{t=1}^{T}(f^{\mathbf{w}_t}(\mathbf{x}_u))^2 - \left(\frac{1}{T}\sum_{t=1}^{T} f^{\mathbf{w}_t}(\mathbf{x}_u)\right)^2$, where the first and the last two terms correspond to aleatoric and epistemic uncertainty respectively. In addition, the variance of each complex-valued pixel is given by the sum of real and imaginary components: $\mathbb{V}[\mathbf{z}] = \mathbb{V}[\mathfrak{R}(\mathbf{z})] + \mathbb{V}[\mathfrak{I}(\mathbf{z})]$.

Network Architectures. We consider UNET [4] and DC-CNN [9] as the base architectures $f^{\mathbf{w}}(\mathbf{x}_u)$. Note that the design of $g^{\mathbf{w}}(\mathbf{x}_u)$ is flexible. In particular, one can independently parametrise f and g, or consider one network with multiple heads. In the former case, $g^{\mathbf{w}}(\mathbf{x}_u)$ models *intrinsic* data uncertainty [10], whereas in the latter case, the uncertainty is correlated with the mean prediction. For DC-CNN, we consider both variants: *DC-CNN1* aggregates the penultimate feature maps from each sub-network, which is fed into a 5-layer variance network. For *DC-CNN2*, an independent 5-layer variance network is trained directly from the undersampled image. For UNET, $f^{\mathbf{w}}(\mathbf{x}_u)$ and $g^{\mathbf{w}}(\mathbf{x}_u)$ share the same encoder but have independent decoders. See Fig. 1 for more details.

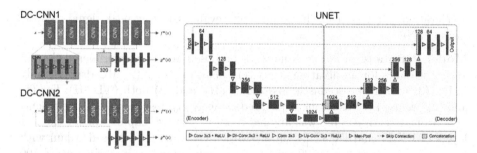

Fig. 1. The proposed network architectures. For DC-CNN1, f and g are correlated whereas for DC-CNN2, f and g are conditionally independent. For UNET, f and g share the same encoder but have two separate decoding paths.

3   Experiments and Results

Dataset: Two datasets were considered for the experiments. *Dataset A* consists of 5000 short-axis cardiac cine MR images from the UK Biobank study [8], which was acquired using bSSFP sequence, matrix size 208×187, 50 frames and a pixel resolution of $1.8 \times 1.8 \times 10.0\,\text{mm}^3$. Since only the magnitude images were available, we simulated the phase components using slowly varying sinusoidal waves. *Dataset B* consists of 10 fully sampled short-axis cardiac cine MR scans acquired at St. Thomas Hospital, UK, using bSSFP sequence with 32-channels, matrix size 192×190, 30 frames, $320 \times 320\,\text{mm}$ FOV and $10\,\text{mm}$ slice thickness. The multi-coil data was recombined into a single complex-valued image using SENSE, which was then treated as the ground truth image. Both datasets were cropped to 192×192.

Experiment Setup: In this work, we investigate the following questions: (1) How do the Bayesian networks perform compared to the standard networks? (2) How do the generated uncertainty maps look like for (a) same dataset, same undersampling scheme, different acceleration factors, (b) same dataset, different undersampling scheme, and (c) different dataset? To answer these questions, the following experimental setting was considered: Dataset A was split into 4000 training subjects and 1000 test subjects. For training, we used 1D Cartesian undersampling, where each line was sampled according to a zero-mean Gaussian distribution. The undersampling masks were generated on-the-fly as we trained, and the acceleration factor was chosen arbitrarily from $n_{\text{acc}} \in [1, 5]$. Note that the networks perform better when they are fine-tuned on a fixed acceleration factor alone. However, for this work, this setup sufficed as we were only interested in the relative performance of the Bayesian formulations. For testing, we used 1000 test subjects from Dataset A and all subjects from Dataset B. In addition, three different undersampling patterns were considered: 1D Cartesian, radial and low-resolution undersampling (SR). We used golden-angle sampling for radial undersampling and for SR, the lowest frequencies were acquired until the desired acceleration factor is met. The results were evaluated using peak signal-to-noise ratio (PSNR).

Model Parameters: For each network proposed above, we considered the following variants for an ablation study: (1) plain network, (2) MC-dropout only (+D), (3) with heteroscedastic loss only (+H), and (4) both (+D+H). For (1) and (2), we used the usual mean squared error (MSE) loss instead. The element-wise dropout with $p = 0.2$ was applied to every feature map except for the last layers of UNET and DC-CNN sub-networks. For training, we used Adam with $\alpha = 10^{-4}, \beta_1 = 0.9, \beta_2 = 0.999$, where α was reduced by a factor of 0.1 every 100 epochs. Each network was trained for 300 epochs, using He initialisation, weight decay of $\lambda = 10^{-6}$ and a mini-batch size 8. For data augmentation, affine transformations were applied on-the-fly, where parameters were sampled from $360°$ rotation, ± 20 pixel shift and scaling factor $s \in [0.9, 1.3]$. For MC-dropout, we used $T = 20$ samples as we empirically found that the result rapidly plateaued beyond that. We used PyTorch for our implementations.

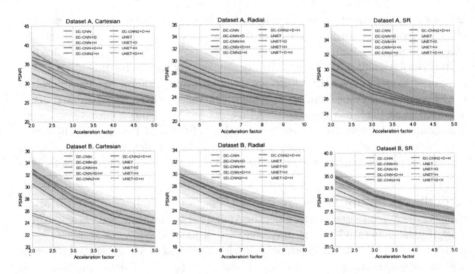

Fig. 2. Quantitative error of all models trained on Dataset A with Cartesian under-sampling for acceleration factor up to 5, tested on different combinations of dataset, undersampling scheme and acceleration factor.

Results: In Fig. 2, the quantitative results are summarised for each dataset and undersampling scheme for a range of acceleration factors (AF). For dataset A with Cartesian undersampling (the closest to the training distribution), the Bayesian methods had poorer performance compared to the baseline networks. However, interestingly, the performance gap was tightened when the experiment was repeated with the different undersampling schemes or dataset B. For DC-CNN, the plain network achieved the highest PSNR and DC-CNN1+D+H performed the poorest. This might be either because the variance estimate may be too noisy during the training due to dropout, or being stuck in a suboptimal local minimum as a result of f and g competing. For UNET, the Bayesian models consistently outperformed the baseline for dataset B. This suggests that the proposed Bayesian formulation could alleviate the network overfitting a specific distribution when the model is over-parametrised.

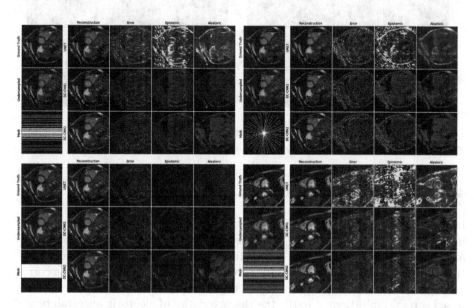

Fig. 3. Visualisation of the generated uncertainty maps for different undersampling patterns and datasets. *(top left)* Dataset A, Cartesian, AF = 3 *(top right)* Dataset A, radial, AF = 8 *(bottom left)* Dataset A, SR, AF = 3, *(bottom right)* Dataset B, Cartesian, AF = 3. Note that the error and uncertainty maps are normalised across the figure.

The generated epistemic and aleatoric uncertainty maps for UNET+D+H, DC-CNN1+D+H and DC-CNN2+D+H are displayed in Fig. 3. We see that, in terms of scale, there is a rough correlation between the error map and the epistemic uncertainty map. However, when each uncertainty map is inspected in detail, they do not necessarily highlight the regions with highest error. For aleatoric uncertainty, it tends to highlight image borders, but they do not consistently correspond to the most aliased regions of the undersampled input. In Fig. 4, we compare the epistemic and aleatoric uncertainty maps generated by DC-CNN1+D+H and DC-CNN2+D+H from dataset A with Cartesian undersampling for different AFs. We can see that for DC-CNN1, the uncertainty level increased as AF was increased. For DC-CNN2, we can observe a higher level of uncertainty across the image, where the edges are highlighted more dominantly. We note that the observations made here are consistent with literature [10].

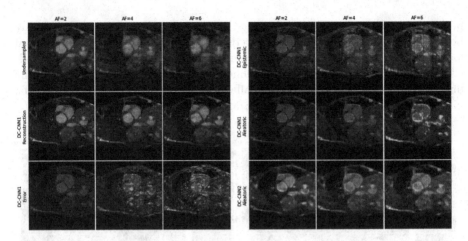

Fig. 4. Visualisation of epistemic and aleatoric uncertainty generated by DC-CNN1 and DC-CNN2 overlaid on the ground-truth image

4   Discussion and Conclusion

In this work, we evaluated MC-dropout and heteroscedastic loss for the MR image reconstruction problem. We observed that the Bayesian methods performed competitively when the data is further away from the training distribution and the generated epistemic and aleatoric uncertainty maps showed a correlation with the error maps. However, we note that the current form of modelling posed several limitations. Firstly, the characteristics of aleatoric uncertainty are heavily dependant on whether f and g are correlated or not, an architectural decision that has to be made by the users based on task-oriented goals. Secondly, we also noticed that between the generated error and the uncertainty maps, there were noticeable discrepancies at fine-scale. For epistemic uncertainty map, we speculate that this may be because MC-dropout is a simple technique and cannot capture the full model uncertainty for the reconstruction networks. For aleatoric uncertainty map, it is presumably because the proposed methods model only pixel-wise uncertainty (i.e. only the diagonal entries of the covariance matrix). We hypothesize that such simplification is a poor approximation for modelling the variance in MR reconstruction, as aliasing caused by random undersampling is distributed across the entire image. A better modelling of such covariance matrix is therefore likely to improve the results. Finally, albeit parallelisable, obtaining epistemic uncertainty requires T forward passes, which may be problematic for real-time applications. Nevertheless, we believe that Bayesian deep learning has a great scope for improvement and is a crucial step towards better characterisation of deep reconstruction networks.

Acknowledgements. Jo Schlemper is partially funded by EPSRC Grant (EP/P001009/1).

References

1. Cohen, J.P., Luck, M., Honari, S.: Distribution matching losses can hallucinate features in medical image translation. arXiv preprint arXiv:1805.08841 (2018)
2. Gal, Y.: Uncertainty in deep learning. University of Cambridge (2016)
3. Hammernik, K., et al.: Learning a variational network for reconstruction of accelerated MRI data. Magn. Reson. Med. **79**, 3055–3071 (2017)
4. Han, Y., Yoo, J., Kim, H.H., Shin, H.J., Sung, K., Ye, J.C.: Deep learning with domain adaptation for accelerated projection-reconstruction MR. Magn. Reson. Med. **80**(3), 1189–1205 (2018)
5. Kendall, A., Gal, Y.: What uncertainties do we need in Bayesian deep learning for computer vision? In: Advances in Neural Information Processing Systems, pp. 5580–5590 (2017)
6. Knoll, F., Hammernik, K., Kobler, E., Pock, T., Recht, M.P., Sodickson, D.K.: Assessment of the generalization of learned image reconstruction and the potential for transfer learning. Magn. Reson. Med. (2018)
7. Mardani, M., et al.: Deep generative adversarial networks for compressed sensing automates MRI. arXiv preprint arXiv:1706.00051 (2017)
8. Petersen, S.E., et al.: UK Biobank's cardiovascular magnetic resonance protocol. J. Cardiovasc. Magn. Reson. **18**(1), 8 (2016). Feb
9. Schlemper, J., Caballero, J., Hajnal, J.V., Price, A., Rueckert, D.: A deep cascade of convolutional neural networks for dynamic MR image reconstruction. IEEE Trans. Med. Imaging **37** (2017)
10. Tanno, R., Ghosh, A., Grussu, F., Kaden, E., Criminisi, A., Alexander, D.C.: Bayesian image quality transfer. In: Ourselin, S., Joskowicz, L., Sabuncu, M.R., Unal, G., Wells, W. (eds.) MICCAI 2016 Part II. LNCS, vol. 9901, pp. 265–273. Springer, Cham (2016). https://doi.org/10.1007/978-3-319-46723-8_31
11. Tezcan, K.C., Baumgartner, C.F., Konukoglu, E.: MR image reconstruction using the learned data distribution as prior. CoRR abs/1711.11386 (2017). http://arxiv.org/abs/1711.11386
12. Yang, G., et al.: DAGAN: deep de-aliasing generative adversarial networks for fast compressed sensing MRI reconstruction. IEEE Trans. Med. Imaging **37**(6), 1310–1321 (2018)
13. Ye, J.C., Han, Y., Cha, E.: Deep convolutional framelets: a general deep learning framework for inverse problems. SIAM J. Imaging Sci. **11**(2), 991–1048 (2018)

Deep Learning for Computed Tomography

Sparse-View CT Reconstruction Using Wasserstein GANs

Franz Thaler[1(✉)], Kerstin Hammernik[1], Christian Payer[1], Martin Urschler[2], and Darko Štern[1,2]

[1] Institute of Computer Graphics and Vision, Graz University of Technology, Graz, Austria
f.thaler@student.tugraz.at, stern@icg.tugraz.at
[2] Ludwig Boltzmann Institute for Clinical Forensic Imaging, Graz, Austria

Abstract. We propose a 2D computed tomography (CT) slice image reconstruction method from a limited number of projection images using Wasserstein generative adversarial networks (wGAN). Our wGAN optimizes the 2D CT image reconstruction by utilizing an adversarial loss to improve the perceived image quality as well as an L_1 content loss to enforce structural similarity to the target image. We evaluate our wGANs using different weight factors between the two loss functions and compare to a convolutional neural network (CNN) optimized on L_1 and the Filtered Backprojection (FBP) method. The evaluation shows that the results generated by the machine learning based approaches are substantially better than those from the FBP method. In contrast to the blurrier looking images generated by the CNNs trained on L_1, the wGANs results appear sharper and seem to contain more structural information. We show that a certain amount of projection data is needed to get a correct representation of the anatomical correspondences.

Keywords: Computed tomography · Sparse-view reconstruction
Convolutional neural networks · Generative adversarial networks
L1 loss

1 Introduction

Computed tomography (CT) is a non-invasive image modality to visualize the interior body structure, enabling fast acquisition and high image quality. To generate a three dimensional (3D) CT image, multiple 2D X-ray projection images of the subject are acquired from different angles on the axial plane and used for reconstruction. The Filtered Backprojection (FBP) is a well established method for 3D CT reconstruction. However, the quality of the reconstructed image using FBP heavily depends on the number of projection images, which correlates to the amount of ionizing radiation exposed.

This work was supported by the Austrian Science Fund (FWF): P28078-N33 and by the Austrian Science Fund (FWF) under the START project BIVISION, No. Y729.

© Springer Nature Switzerland AG 2018
F. Knoll et al. (Eds.): MLMIR 2018, LNCS 11074, pp. 75–82, 2018.
https://doi.org/10.1007/978-3-030-00129-2_9

As the risk of cancer is increased by radiation exposure, different approaches exist to decrease the radiation dose. Two popular approaches to decrease radiation dose are tube current reduction, resulting in degraded image quality, and beam blocking, which restricts the amount of X-rays reaching the subject in a physical way, resulting in streaking artifacts. Recent promising results for ionizing dose reduction were achieved by utilizing convolutional neural networks (CNN) [3,4,13] and made deep learning also attractive for image reconstruction.

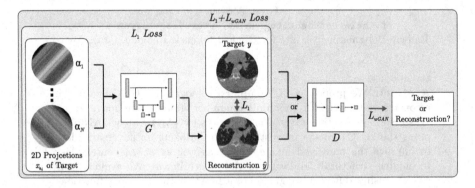

Fig. 1. Reconstruction $\hat{y}$ of a target image y from a limited number of 2D projection images x_{α_i} generated from y with different angles α_i using a combination of a wGAN loss L_{wGAN} and an additional content loss L_1. The generator G is based on the U-Net [7], the discriminator D results in a single scalar value.

Reducing the number of X-ray image views acquired and used for CT reconstruction is another approach to decrease the amount of radiation exposed. Sparse-view CT reconstruction becomes important during minimally invasive and image guided surgeries, where multiple X-ray images are acquired repeatedly during intervention to precisely locate the instruments, leading to an exposure to ionizing radiation for both the patient and medical staff. In a recent CNN based approach [10], residual learning is used to extract the artifacts from the FBP image which are then subtracted from the FBP image to obtain the clean reconstruction. In contrast to other CNN based approaches that learn the transformation from a low quality, FBP based reconstructed CT image to a high quality CT image, in our previous work [9], we learned a direct mapping from 3D digitally reconstructed radiographs (DRR) to the full 3D CT reconstruction using a U-Net architecture. However, the downside of this approach is that the reconstructed images look blurry due to the used L_1 loss. This observation suggests to improve on the loss function used for training.

Generative adverserial networks (GANs), which can generate realistically looking images, have a great potential to improve also the reconstruction quality of medical images. A GAN requires two networks to be trained: a generator, which has the goal to create images coming from a target distribution, and a discriminator, which has to distinguish between the generated and the real target

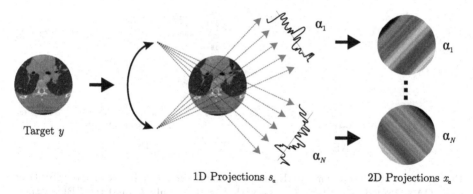

Fig. 2. Generation of 1D projections s_α from a target 2D CT slice image y for a number of N fixed angles α_i. All s_α are further processed by repeating in the direction of the respective α yielding the 2D projection images x_α used as network input.

distribution. However, GANs are inherently hard to train and often suffer from stability issues. Wasserstein GANs (wGANs) [1], which were further improved by utilizing a gradient penalty [2], provide a way to stabilize the training. Combined with a content loss such as L_1, state-of-the-art results were achieved for super resolution [5] and in medical imaging [6,8,11,12].

However, as GANs were initially proposed to generate new images from noise, its applicability to medical applications is an open question. In this work, we want to gain insights in the applicability of wGANs for improving the image quality for 2D CT image slice reconstruction from a limited number of projection images. We investigate the role of an additional content loss for improved reconstruction quality and provide insights in the amount of projection images that are necessary for anatomically correct reconstructions.

2 Method

In our deep learning based method we utilize wGANs with gradient penalty in combination with a content loss L_1 to improve the reconstruction of 2D axial CT slices, see Fig. 1. Our method is trained to reconstruct the target 2D CT axial slice directly from a small number of 2D projection images generated by extending 1D projections of the target image, see Fig. 2.

Projection Image Generation: We generated a 1D sum projection s_{α_i} from a target 2D axial CT slice $y \in Y$ for different angles $\alpha_i, i \in \{1, \dots, N\}$, see Fig. 2. The angles α are uniformly distributed in the range of $0°$ to $180°$ with a fixed angle between them. With the same size as y, the 2D projection image x_{α_i} is generated by repeating s_{α_i} in the direction of α_i.

wGAN Architecture: Based on the U-Net [7], the generator G of wGAN uses a set of 2D projection images x_α to generate a 2D image $\hat{y} \in \hat{Y}$, which is as similar as possible to $y \in Y$. Alternately receiving an image from Y and $\hat{Y}$,

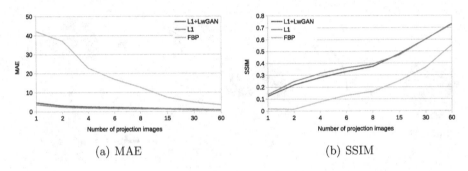

(a) MAE   (b) SSIM

Fig. 3. Mean absolute error (MAE) and structural similarity index metric (SSIM) of our wGAN trained using $L_1 + L_{wGAN}$ with $\lambda = 10^{-3}$, only L_1 and the FBP method compared to the ground truth for a different number of projection images

the task of the discriminator D of wGAN is to recognize from which of these two distributions the currently observed image is coming. The architecture of D consists of consecutive 2D convolution layers and 2D max pooling layers, which are followed by a fully connected layer resulting in a single scalar value.

Loss Functions: The discriminator's loss is defined as

$$L_D = -D(y) + D(\hat{y}) + \rho, \tag{1}$$

where $D(y)$ is the discriminator's predicted probability for y coming from Y, $D(\hat{y})$ is the predicted probability for $\hat{y}$ coming also from Y and ρ is the gradient penalty, which is used to stabilize the training of the wGAN [2].

The generator's loss is defined as

$$L_G = L_1 - \lambda \cdot D(\hat{y}) = L_1 + \lambda \cdot L_{wGAN}, \tag{2}$$

where λ is used as a weight between the adversarial loss $L_{wGAN} = -D(\hat{y})$ and L_1 loss, which is defined as

$$L_1 = \frac{1}{|M|} \sum_{m \in M} |\hat{y}_m - y_m|, \tag{3}$$

where $m \in M$ are corresponding pixels in $\hat{y}$ and y, and M is the set of all pixels.

2.1 Experimental Setup

Our data set consists of 10 3D CT images containing information from neck to pelvis. To decrease the training time, we downsampled the axial slices for all images to a size of 128×128. We separated the 3D CT images into eight training and two testing images. During training, the 2D target image is selected as a random axial slice from a training 3D CT image that is augmented on the fly by random translation, rotation and scaling coming from a uniform distribution. To prevent the problem of different amounts of image data present in projection

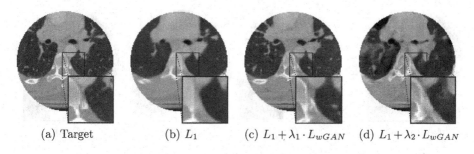

(a) Target   (b) L_1 (c) $L_1 + \lambda_1 \cdot L_{wGAN}$ (d) $L_1 + \lambda_2 \cdot L_{wGAN}$

Fig. 4. The target compared to reconstruction results for eight projections generated by L_1 and $L_1 + L_{wGAN}$ with two different values for λ. $\lambda_1 = 10^{-3}$ (default), $\lambda_2 = 10^{-1}$.

images from different angles when generated from a square shaped target image, all targets are masked by a circle. We used the same mask when the loss is calculated. We experiment with a different number $N = \{1, 2, 4, 6, 8, 15, 30, 60\}$ of projection images used for reconstruction of 2D CT axial slice images. The results are compared quantitatively to the FBP method by calculating the mean absolute error (MAE) and the structural similarity index metric (SSIM). When results are compared qualitatively, all images share the same brightness setting, but some values are truncated to give a better contrast.

All networks were trained using a mini-batch size of 16 and 80.000 iterations, while the discriminator was trained five times for each iteration. We used Adam as an optimizer for all networks with a learning rate of 0.0001, $\beta_1 = 0.5$ and $\beta_2 = 0.9$. We used a four level deep U-Net [7] as our generator. For both the generator and the discriminator we used a kernel size of 3×3 and 64 intermediate convolutional filters. As activation function, we used ReLU for the generator and Leaky ReLU for the discriminator.

3   Results

Our results for a different number of projection images used for reconstruction of 2D CT axial slice images are presented quantitatively as MAE in Fig. 3(a) and as SSIM in Fig. 3(b). Qualitative results using eight projection images and a different weight factor λ are shown in Fig. 4. For a different number $N \in \{2, 15, 60\}$ of projection images, Fig. 5 shows the qualitative results for the FBP method and Fig. 6 for using only L_1 loss ($\lambda = 0$) and $L_1 + L_{wGAN}$ loss ($\lambda = 10^{-3}$).

4   Discussion and Conclusion

In this work we investigated the potential use of wGANs for sparse-view CT slice reconstruction, which is motivated by a reduction of ionizing radiation exposure to the patient. While a content loss L_1 enforces similarity to the target image, our U-net based CNN is optimized using a combination of the L_1 and an adversarial

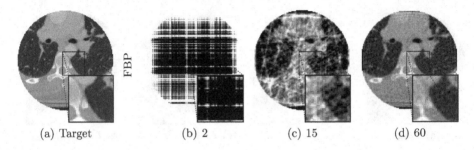

(a) Target   (b) 2   (c) 15   (d) 60

Fig. 5. The target image (a) compared to reconstruction results generated by the FBP method for two (b), 15 (c) and 60 (d) projection images.

loss L_{wGAN} (Eq. (2)) to reconstruct more realistically looking images. In contrast to other machine learning based approaches in which the reconstruction of a high quality CT image is learned from the previously reconstructed low quality CT image [3,4,13], in our approach the CNN learns the reconstruction directly from a limited number of projection images, see Fig. 1.

When a different number of projection images is used to train our CNNs, our quantitative results show that the learning based methods perform substantially better than the FBP, see Fig. 3, which is to be expected, since the FBP does not utilize any prior knowledge in contrast to the CNN based approaches. In terms of the MAE, the CNN trained on L_1-only performs slightly better than the wGAN trained on the combination of L_1 and adversarial loss ($L_1 + L_{wGAN}$). This was expected, since L_1 loss is optimized to minimize MAE. By comparing the SSIM results, we can see that the CNN trained on L_1-only gives better results up to eight projection images, but from that point on the results from L_1-only and $L_1 + L_{wGAN}$ can be considered equal. Although the quantitative results indicate that the CNNs trained on L_1-only provide a better reconstruction than on $L_1 + L_{wGAN}$, they have to be considered with caution, since MAE and SSIM do not represent the human perception of image quality well.

When training CNNs on L_1-only loss using a sparse number of projection images, the qualitative results show that the reconstructed image is blurry without fine structures and clear edges, see Fig. 4(b). Using an additional adversarial loss, the images contain fine structures and clear edges, see Fig. 4(c). However, when the adversarial loss dominates in the loss function, anatomical structures without correspondence to the target image can be introduced, see Fig. 4(d). We investigated the effect of λ by utilizing different orders of magnitude $\lambda = 10^{\{-4,-3,-2,-1,0\}}$ and found $\lambda = 10^{-3}$ to be the optimum. While 10^{-4} leads to results very similar to L_1-only and seemingly without an influence of L_{wGAN}, the results using $10^{\{-2,-1,0\}}$ lead to a clear reduction of structural similarity and thus a loss of anatomical correspondence to the target.

Our results using a different number of projection images in Fig. 5 confirm that the FBP method is not able to produce clinically meaningful images without a proper number of projections. On the other side, our machine learning based approach is able to reconstruct the main anatomical structures of the target

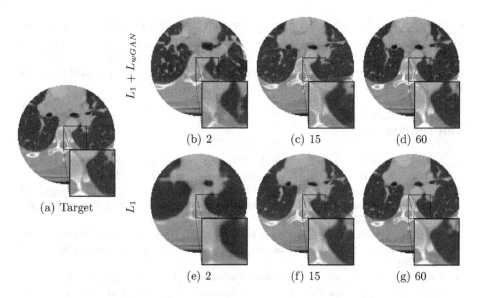

Fig. 6. The target image (a) compared to reconstruction results generated by $L_1 + L_{wGAN}$ with $\lambda = 10^{-3}$ (b, c and d) as well as by L_1 (e, f and g) for two (b, e), 15 (c, f) and 60 (d, g) projection images.

image already from two projection images, see Fig. 6. While using L_1-only loss generates images that give the impression of a heavily blurred target image, the reconstructed image by $L_1 + L_{wGAN}$ loss looks optically more realistic. However, for both reconstructions, the anatomical structures do not always correspond to the target due to a huge amount of missing information making them unsuitable for use in clinical practice. In our experiments we found that 15 projection images are sufficient for our CNN based approaches to achieve a qualitatively good reconstruction. However, the results generated by $L_1 + L_{wGAN}$ are sharper and give more textural information compared to L_1-only loss. The results generated from 60 projection images provide a similar amount of fine details as the target image. Nevertheless, the $L_1 + L_{wGAN}$ result is still slightly sharper than L_1-only loss, especially the fine details in the lung region are visible.

We showed that the combination of an adversarial loss L_{wGAN} and a content loss L_1 improves the visual reconstruction quality. The reconstructions using $L_1 + L_{wGAN}$ appear sharper and more structured compared to the CNN results trained on L_1-only. However, the tradeoff λ is crucial to reduce the amount of newly introduced information by the wGAN and guide the reconstruction in a direction close to the target image. While images generated by the CNNs trained on L_1-only appear blurry, the additional information present in the wGAN results trained on $L_1 + L_{wGAN}$ can potentially lead to misinterpretation in a clinical relevant context if not enough data is available for reconstruction.

In conclusion, the wGANs have a potential to improve the perceived image quality even from a huge amount of missing information, however, it is dependent on the application and domain, whether the kind of artifacts introduced are tolerable, which is an open question in medical imaging. To further evaluate anatomical correspondence, in our future work we will validate the perceived image quality of our approach by expert radiologists and also compare to other state-of-the-art methods based on compressed sensing.

References

1. Arjovsky, M., Chintala, S., Bottou, L.: Wasserstein generative adversarial networks. In: International Conference on Machine Learning, pp. 214–223 (2017)
2. Gulrajani, I., Ahmed, F., Arjovsky, M., Dumoulin, V., Courville, A.C.: Improved training of Wasserstein GANs. In: Advances in Neural Information Processing Systems, pp. 5769–5779 (2017)
3. Jin, K.H., McCann, M.T., Froustey, E., Unser, M.: Deep convolutional neural network for inverse problems in imaging. IEEE Trans. Image Process. **26**(9), 4509–4522 (2017)
4. Kang, E., Min, J., Ye, J.C.: A deep convolutional neural network using directional wavelets for low-dose X-ray CT reconstruction. Med. Phys. **44**(10), e360–e375 (2017)
5. Ledig, C., et al.: Photo-realistic single image super-resolution using a generative adversarial network. In: Proceedings of the IEEE Conference on Computer Vision and Pattern Recognition, pp. 4681–4690 (2017)
6. Mardani, M., et al.: Deep generative adversarial networks for compressed sensing automates MRI. Preprint arXiv:1706.00051 (2017)
7. Ronneberger, O., Fischer, P., Brox, T.: U-Net: convolutional networks for biomedical image segmentation. In: Navab, N., Hornegger, J., Wells, W.M., Frangi, A.F. (eds.) MICCAI 2015 Part III. LNCS, vol. 9351, pp. 234–241. Springer, Cham (2015). https://doi.org/10.1007/978-3-319-24574-4_28
8. Seitzer, M., et al.: Adversarial and perceptual refinement for compressed sensing MRI reconstruction. Accepted at International Conference on Medical Image Computing and Computer-Assisted Intervention (2018)
9. Thaler, F., Payer, C., Štern, D.: Volumetric reconstruction from a limited number of digitally reconstructed radiographs using CNNs. In: Proceedings of the OAGM Workshop 2018, pp. 13–19. Verlag der TU Graz (2018)
10. Xie, S., et al.: Artifact removal using improved GoogLeNet for sparse-view CT reconstruction. Sci. Rep. **8**(1), 6700 (2018)
11. Yang, G., et al.: Dagan: deep de-aliasing generative adversarial networks for fast compressed sensing MRI reconstruction. IEEE Trans. Med. Imaging **37**(6), 1310–1321 (2018)
12. Yang, Q., et al.: Low-dose CT image denoising using a generative adversarial network with Wasserstein distance and perceptual loss. IEEE Trans. Med. Imaging **37**(6), 1348–1357 (2018)
13. Yang, X., et al.: Low-dose X-ray tomography through a deep convolutional neural network. Sci. Rep. **8**(1), 2575 (2018)

Detecting Anatomical Landmarks for Motion Estimation in Weight-Bearing Imaging of Knees

Bastian Bier[1]([✉]), Katharina Aschoff[1], Christopher Syben[1], Mathias Unberath[2], Marc Levenston[3], Garry Gold[3], Rebecca Fahrig[3], and Andreas Maier[1]

[1] Pattern Recognition Lab, Friedrich-Alexander-Universität Erlangen-Nürnberg,
Erlangen, Germany
bastian.bier@fau.de
[2] Laboratory for Computational Sensing and Robotics,
Johns Hopkins University, Baltimore, USA
[3] Radiological Sciences Laboratory, Stanford University, Stanford, USA

Abstract. Patient motion is one of the major challenges in cone-beam computed tomography (CBCT) scans acquired under weight-bearing conditions, since it leads to severe artifacts in reconstructions. In knee imaging, a state-of-the-art approach to compensate for patient motion uses fiducial markers attached to the skin. However, marker placement is a tedious and time consuming procedure for both, the physician and the patient. In this manuscript we investigate the use of anatomical landmarks in an attempt to replace externally attached fiducial markers. To this end, we devise a method to automatically detect anatomical landmarks in projection domain X-ray images irrespective of the viewing direction. To overcome the need for annotation of every X-ray image and to assure consistent annotation across images from the same subject, annotations and projection images are generated from 3D CT data. Twelve landmarks are annotated in supine CBCT reconstructions of the knee joint and then propagated to synthetically generated projection images. Then, a sequential Convolutional Neuronal Network is trained to predict the desired landmarks in projection images. The network is evaluated on synthetic images and real clinical data. On synthetic data promising results are achieved with a mean prediction error of 8.4 ± 8.2 pixel. The network generalizes to real clinical data without the need of re-training. However, practical issues, such as the second leg entering the field of view, limit the performance of the method at this stage. Nevertheless, our results are promising and encourage further investigations on the use of anatomical landmarks for motion management.

1 Introduction

C-arm cone-beam computed tomography (CBCT) systems have been used recently to acquire 3D images of the human knee joint under weight-bearing conditions [1,2]. Scans under weight-bearing conditions can be beneficial for the

© Springer Nature Switzerland AG 2018
F. Knoll et al. (Eds.): MLMIR 2018, LNCS 11074, pp. 83–90, 2018.
https://doi.org/10.1007/978-3-030-00129-2_10

investigation of the knee health since it has been shown that the human knee joint shows different properties in a natural position under load compared to a supine acquisition [3]. Load bearing imaging requires dedicated imaging protocols. Using robotic C-arm systems driven in horizontal trajectories [1,4,5], it takes several seconds to acquire enough 2D projection images for a clinically satisfying reconstruction. During that time, the standing patient might move involuntarily. This motion leads to inconsistencies in the projection data, and thus, to motion artifacts in the reconstructions. Therefore, motion compensation is indispensable for achieving diagnostic reconstruction quality in weight-bearing CBCT of the knee.

In order to reduce motion induced artifacts in such scenarios, various approaches have been proposed: autofocus-based methods optimize image-quality criteria in reconstructions [6], registration-based approaches align acquired images to a static reference [4,7,8], while range camera-based solutions image the knee surface to estimate patient motion [5]. Another state-of-the-art method uses metallic fiducial markers externally attached to the skin of the knee [1,4]. Due to their high attenuation, these markers are easily visible and detectable in the 2D projections. Using the detected marker locations, 3D reference marker positions can be computed. Having 2D positions as well as corresponding 3D reference positions, a refined C-arm trajectory can be computed analytically in a 2D/3D alignment step, i.e. without the need for computation-heavy optimization. Despite best-in-class performance, the usability of this method suffers: marker placement is time consuming, interrupts the clinical workflow, and must be executed carefully since markers must not overlap in the projections. Therefore, a purely image-based method similar to the fiducial marker-based approach is desirable.

A promising candidate to replace the markers are anatomical landmarks visible in projection images. Finding key points and establishing correspondences in images of the same scene is a well understood concept in computer vision. However, this concept does not translate easily to transmission imaging, where the appearance of the same landmark can vary tremendously dependent on the viewing direction. Recently, Convolutional Neuronal Network (CNN)-based sequential predication frameworks have shown promising performance in detecting anatomical landmarks in X-ray transmission images of the pelvis across a large range of viewing angles of the C-arm CT system [9].

Here, we transfer the work in Bier and Unberath *et al.* [9] to view-independent anatomical landmark detection in CBCT short scans of knees under weight-bearing conditions. To this end, a CNN is trained on synthetic projection images generated from 3D CBCT data. In total, twelve anatomical landmarks are manually annotated in 3D and then predicted in projection domain. The network readily establishes landmark correspondence across images suggesting that sufficiently accurate landmark detection will pave the way for "anatomical marker"-based motion compensation. Our landmark detection is evaluated on a simulated short scan, and two clinical CBCT scans in supine and weight-bearing condition, respectively. The network is trained on synthetic data [9], yet, generalizes to real projection images without the need of re-training.

2   Method

2.1   X-Ray Invariant Anatomical Landmark Detection

Detection of anatomical landmarks irrespective of the viewing direction has been proposed recently [9]. The concept of landmark detection was derived from a sequential prediction framework, namely the Convolutional Pose Machine (CPM) [10]. This network architecture was initially developed to detect human joint positions in RGB images and provides key benefits: it combines local image features with increasingly refined belief maps to establish landmark relationships. The network processes each image independently and, for each landmark, predicts a belief map indicating the landmark position.

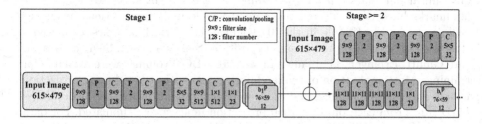

Fig. 1. Network architecture [9]

The network involves successive processing of the input image over several stages, see Fig. 1. In the first stage, the network architecture consists of convolutional and pooling layers, which result in initial belief maps. In the following stages, these belief maps are refined using both local image features and the belief maps of the previous stage. The cost function of the network is the difference between the predicted belief maps b_t^p and the ground truth belief maps b_t^* of all landmarks $p \in \{1, .., P\}$ and in each stage t: consequently, the l_2 norm of this difference defines the cost function f_t [10]:

$$f_t = \sum_{p=1}^{P} \|b_t^p - b_t^*\|_2^2. \tag{1}$$

This network structure has several properties: it has a large receptive field (160 × 160 pixels) on the input image, empowering the network to learn characteristic global configurations over long-distances. The stage-wise manner also allows the network to resolve ambiguities due to similar local appearance. Further, accumulating the loss after each stage prevents vanishing gradients that often occur in large CNNs [10].

2.2   Training

In order to train the network, projection images and corresponding landmark positions have to be known. We follow the approach discussed in [9,11] and

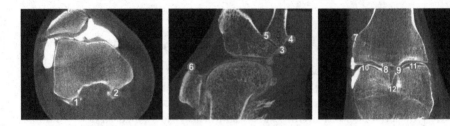

Fig. 2. Anatomical landmarks defined on the surface of the bones in the knee joint

generate projection images and annotations synthetically by annotating twelve anatomical landmarks in CBCT volumes of the human knee, see Fig. 2. The landmarks have been selected to be good visible in the projections images as well as clearly identifiable in the 3D volume. The CBCT volumes were reconstructions of scans acquired in supine position (Siemens Zeego, Siemens Healthcare GmbH, Erlangen, Germany). In total 16 CBCT volumes were available for training. After annotation of the landmark positions in the volumes, projection images and corresponding annotations were generated synthetically using CON-RAD [12]. From each dataset, 1000 projection images were simulated. For data augmentation purposes, images were sampled during projection generation on a spherical segment with a range of 240° LAO/RAO and 20° in CRAN/CAUD. This range covers more than the necessary variance of a common CBCT short scan. Additionally, random translations in three Cartesian axes and horizontal flipping of the projections were used. The belief map of a particular landmark consists of a single normal distribution centered at the true landmark location. The size of the projections was 615 × 479 with a pixel size of 0.6 mm. The belief maps were downsampled eight times.

16 supine CT scans, split 14 × 1 × 1-fold in training, validation and testing data are used for the training and testing. The network was trained with six stages for 30 epochs with a constant learning rate of 0.00001 and a batch size of one. The optimization was done using Adam optimization. Figure 3 shows that convergence is reached during both training and validation.

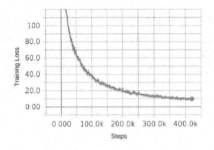
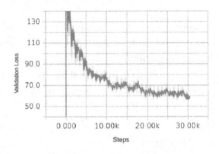

Fig. 3. Training loss (left side) and Validation loss (right side)

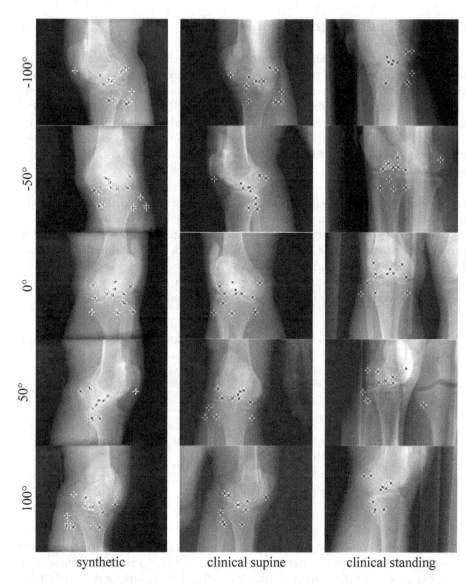

Fig. 4. Detection results on the synthetic (left), a supine scan (center), and a standing scan (right)

2.3 Landmark Estimation

The network outputs twelve belief maps that indicate the landmark positions. The belief map after each step is accumulated, and the 2D landmark position is defined as the maximum response in the accumulated belief map.

3 Experiments and Results

Landmark detection is evaluated quantitatively on a synthetic short scan dataset as well as qualitatively on two clinical CBCT scans in supine and standing condition, respectively. In order to investigate the prediction results over the complete trajectory, detection results sampled from different directions are represented in Fig. 4. Column-wise from left to right, we show results on the synthetic dataset, the real clinical data in supine and in standing conditions, respectively. Detected landmarks are highlighted in red and reference marker positions in white, wherever available.

The detection results on the synthetic dataset are in good agreement with the ground truth label positions. Visually, also the detected landmarks in the real clinical images are in agreement with the labeled locations. Note that in the supine scan also a part of the patient's feet is present in some parts of the projections. However, this does not seem to influence the landmark detections. In the projections acquired under weight-bearing conditions a second leg is also present in parts of the projection. Since there is a second knee in the field of view, the detection of the landmarks is not consistently on one leg only.

Table 1. Average distance [pixels] of the predicted landmarks to the ground truth location

Landmark #	Distance ($\mu \pm \sigma$)	Landmark #	Distance ($\mu \pm \sigma$)
1	6.6 ± 2.0	7	17.7 ± 8.6
2	10.5 ± 3.9	8	3.2 ± 1.9
3	3.8 ± 1.4	9	5.1 ± 1.6
4	8.7 ± 2.5	10	5.1 ± 1.6
5	9.5 ± 5.0	11	7.0 ± 4.6
6	18.1 ± 19.2	12	5.7 ± 3.9

Since the reference landmark locations were known on the synthetic short scan dataset, we computed the average distance to the ground truth landmark locations as well as the detection rate. We define a landmark as detected, if the distance to its ground truth location is <15 pixel and the maximum belief is ≥0.4. The average distance of the landmark detections on the simulated short scan was then 8.4±8.2 pixels and a detection accuracy of 89.16% is reached. Furthermore, we investigated the quality of the selected anatomical landmarks and computed the average distance for each landmark. The results of this are shown in Table 1. Large differences between individual landmarks can be observed here. The best landmarks are the tip of the Fibula (landmark #3) and landmarks inside the knee joint. It is further noticeable that landmarks with less other neighboring landmarks, e.g. on the Patella (landmark #6), or on the Tibia (landmark #7), are detected with a much higher uncertainty.

4 Conclusion and Outlook

The presence of patient motion during CBCT scans is one of the major challenges in CBCT acquisitions acquired under weight-bearing conditions. Currently, an approach based on metallic fiducial markers is used to estimate motion. However, marker placement is time consuming and tedious. Therefore, we investigated the feasibility of using anatomical landmarks as image-based markers instead.

An X-ray invariant anatomical landmark detection approach was utilized to detect landmarks in projection images. Trained on high quality supine data of the knee, the network predicted belief maps in which the position of the anatomical landmarks can be estimated in synthetic as well as in real clinical data. These landmarks could be used to estimate motion using a 2D/3D based registration approach. The estimation of the motion with these detections is subject of future work. It also had been shown that some landmarks could be estimated more robustly than others. This might contain the potential to incorporate this information in the further processing steps. Furthermore, we believe that such approaches might be applicable to compensate other complex body motion [13], e. g., using motion models for respiratory [14] or cardiac motion [15].

Despite promising results on projection images of the knee, some limitations remain. The large angular range of short scans unavoidably implies the presence of both legs in the field of view. On the one hand, bones superimpose and hinder the detection. On the other hand, we observed "jumping" of detections from one knee to the other. These observations further motivate why landmark detection seems to visually perform better on supine than on standing data. Moreover, the method results in limited accuracy due to downsampling of the ground truth belief maps by factor of around eight. To improve the accuracy, an advanced network incorporating skip-ahead-connections might increase the performance.

Despite these limitations, this work shows that the automatically landmark detection works well for synthetically generated as well as for real X-ray projection images of knee joints. In future work, we will investigate methods to make landmark prediction more robust, particularly in presence of additional anatomy, and to use our predictions to estimate and compensate for patient motion during reconstruction.

References

1. Choi, J., et al.: Fiducial marker-based correction for involuntary motion in weight-bearing C-arm CT scanning of knees Part I. Numerical model-based optimization. Med. Phys. **41**(6), 061902 (2014)
2. Choi, J.H., et al.: Fiducial marker-based correction for involuntary motion in weight-bearing C-arm CT scanning of knees II. Experiment. Med. Phys. **41**(6), 061902 (2014)
3. Powers, C.M., Ward, S.R., Fredericson, M.: Knee extension in persons with lateral subluxation of the patella : a preliminary study. J. Orthop. Sports Phys. Ther. **33**(11), 677–685 (2013)

4. Berger, M., et al.: Marker-free motion correction in weight-bearing cone-beam CT of the knee joint. Med. Phys. **43**(3), 1235–1248 (2016)
5. Bier, B., et al.: Range imaging for motion compensation in C-arm cone-beam CT of knees under weight-bearing conditions. J. Imaging **4**(4), 561–570 (2018)
6. Sisniega, A., Stayman, J., Yorkston, J., Siewerdsen, J., Zbijewski, W.: Motion compensation in extremity cone-beam CT using a penalized image sharpness criterion. Phys. Med. Biol. **62**(9), 3712–3734 (2017)
7. Unberath, M., Choi, J.H., Berger, M., Maier, A., Fahrig, R.: Image-based compensation for involuntary motion in weight-bearing C-arm cone-beam CT scanning of knees. In: SPIE Medical Imaging, vol. 9413, March 2015. 94130D
8. Ouadah, S., Jacobson, M., Stayman, J.W., Ehtiati, T., Weiss, C., Siewerdsen, J.H.: Correction of patient motion in cone-beam CT Correction of patient motion in cone-beam CT using 3D 2D registration. Phys. Med. Biol. **62**, 8813–8831 (2017)
9. Bier, B., et al.: X-ray-transform invariant anatomical landmark detection for pelvic trauma surgery. In: International Conference on Medical Image Computing and Computer-Assisted Intervention. Springer (2018 to appear)
10. Wei, S.E., Ramakrishna, V., Kanade, T., Sheikh, Y.: Convolutional pose machines. In: CVPR, pp. 4724–4732 (2016)
11. Unberath, M., et al.: DeepDRR-a catalyst for machine learning in fluoroscopy-guided procedures. In: International Conference on Medical Image Computing and Computer-Assisted Intervention. Springer (2018 to appear)
12. Maier, A., et al.: CONRAD - a software framework for cone-beam imaging in radiology. Med. Phys. **40**(11), 111914 (2013)
13. Müller, K., et al.: Image artefact propagation in motion estimation and reconstruction in interventional cardiac C-arm CT. Phys. Med. Biol. **59**(12), 3121 (2014)
14. Geimer, T., Birlutiu, A., Unberath, M., Taubmann, O., Bert, C., Maier, A.: A Kernel ridge regression model for respiratory motion estimation in radiotherapy. Bildverarbeitung für die Medizin 2017. I, pp. 155–160. Springer, Heidelberg (2017). https://doi.org/10.1007/978-3-662-54345-0_38
15. Unberath, M., Geimer, T., Höhn, J., Achenbach, S., Maier, A.: Myocardial twist from X-ray angiography. In: Maier, A., Deserno, T., Handels, H., Maier-Hein, K.H., Palm, C., Tolxdorff, T. (eds.) Bildverarbeitung für die Medizin 2018 - Algorithmen - Systeme - Anwendungen, pp. 365–370. Springer, Heidelberg (2018). https://doi.org/10.1007/978-3-662-56537-7_91

A U-Nets Cascade for Sparse View Computed Tomography

Andreas Kofler[1]([⊠]), Markus Haltmeier[2], Christoph Kolbitsch[3,4], Marc Kachelrieß[5], and Marc Dewey[1]

[1] Department of Radiology, Charité - Universitätsmedizin Berlin, Berlin, Germany
andreas.kofler@charite.de
[2] Department of Mathematics, University of Innsbruck, Innsbruck, Austria
[3] Physikalisch-Technische Bundesanstalt, Braunschweig and Berlin, Germany
[4] Division of Imaging Sciences and Biomedical Engineering,
King's College London, London, UK
[5] Medical Physics in Radiology, German Cancer Research Center,
Heidelberg, Germany

Abstract. We propose a new convolutional neural network architecture for image reconstruction in sparse view computed tomography. The proposed network consists of a cascade of U-nets and data consistency layers. While the U-nets address the undersampling artifacts, the data consistency layers model the specific scanner geometry and make direct use of measured data. We train the network cascade end-to-end on sparse view cardiac CT images. The proposed network's performance is evaluated according to different quantitative measures and compared to the one of a cascade with fully convolutional neural networks with residual connections and to the one of a single U-net with approximately the same number of trainable parameters. While in both experiments the methods show similar performance in terms of quantitative measures, our proposed U-nets cascade yields superior visual results and better preserves the overall image structure as well as fine diagnostic details, e.g. the coronary arteries. The latter is also confirmed by a statistically significant increase of the Haar-wavelet-based perceptual similarity index measure in all the experiments.

Keywords: Deep learning · Convolutional neural networks
Data consistency · Computed tomography · Sparse sampling

1 Introduction

Sparse data-acquisition protocols are widely used in magnetic resonance imaging (MRI) in order to shorten scanning times. In contrast, in computed tomography (CT), the data acquisition process is fast while reducing radiation exposure is an important clinical issue. One possible way to reduce radiation exposure is to decrease the tube current of the X-ray emitting source. However, the direct consequence is decreased image quality due to higher image noise. In this paper,

© Springer Nature Switzerland AG 2018
F. Knoll et al. (Eds.): MLMIR 2018, LNCS 11074, pp. 91–99, 2018.
https://doi.org/10.1007/978-3-030-00129-2_11

we use a sparse view data-acquisition scheme to reach a significant radiation exposure reduction in CT. This can be achieved by masking the X-ray source at certain angular positions during the rotation of the scanner and therefore preventing some X-rays to pass through the patient. Using standard algorithms, images reconstructed from sparse view data exhibit undersampling structures which are related to the scanner geometry as well as the sub-sampling scheme used for data acquisition.

Recently, deep neural networks have shown to be a promising alternative to current state-of-the-art iterative methods for the reconstruction from heavily undersampled CT data. In particular, the U-net [6] has shown its excellent performance in the restoration of undersampled images in CT and MRI [4]. However, these standard network designs can be viewed as post-processing methods, as the network used to remove the artifacts is the only learned component in the reconstruction pipeline. As a consequence, these methods may lack data consistency. In this paper we propose a new network architecture for the image reconstruction from undersampled data in sparse view CT. Our network structure is inspired by the network cascade developed in [7] and consists of a cascade of convolutional neural networks and data consistency layers which minimize a properly-chosen functional. However, while the approach in [7] is based on the isometry of the full MRI forward operator, our data consistency layer is directly applicable to general inverse problems as well. Furthermore, the fully convolutional neural networks (FCNNs) with residual connections are replaced by U-nets. For different, gradient-descent-like data consistency layers, see [2,3].

1.1   Sparse View Computed Tomography

Here and after we work with the discrete setting. By $\mathbf{x} \in \mathbb{R}^n$ we refer to the vector of size $m \times m$ with $m^2 = n$ as representation of the two-dimensional X-ray attenuation function and write $\mathbf{y} \in \mathbb{R}^d$ for a fully sampled sinogram. Further, we use $\mathbf{R}$ to denote the discretized forward operator of a CT scanner, i.e. the discrete X-ray transform specified by the scanner's geometry. We denote the pseudoinverse of the discretized forward operator by $\mathbf{R}^\dagger$. Note that the continuous form of the Radon transform is injective but not surjective. Therefore, we may assume that the Radon transform $\mathbf{R}$ is sampled sufficiently fine such that the discretized full data operator is injective but not surjective as well. Anyway, the approach presented below works for an arbitrary discrete transform $\mathbf{R} \in \mathbb{R}^{d \times n}$.

Assume the data is measured only for lines corresponding to a subset $I \subset J \triangleq \{1, \ldots, d\}$, where J is the full set of projections. The corresponding discretized sparse data forward operator can be modeled by $\mathbf{R}_I = \mathbf{S}_I \mathbf{R}$, where the sub-sampling operator is given by

$$\mathbf{S}_I \mathbf{y}(i) \triangleq \begin{cases} \mathbf{y}(i) & \text{if } i \in I \\ 0 & \text{if } i \in I^c := J \setminus I. \end{cases} \tag{1}$$

The sparse data image reconstruction problem then consists in recovering the image $\mathbf{x} \in \mathbb{R}^n$ from the set of projections, i.e. we want to solve

$$\mathbf{R}_I \mathbf{x} = \mathbf{y}_I. \tag{2}$$

2   Proposed Network Architecture

In the full data case, (2) can be be solved by filtered back-projection, which is a stable numerical implementation of $\mathbf{R}^\dagger$. However, in the sparse view case we have $|I| \ll |I^c|$ and the application of $\mathbf{R}^\dagger$ to data $\mathbf{y}_I$ yields images with severe artifacts. Images with diagnostic quality can usually be obtained by iterative reconstruction methods designed for minimizing $\mathcal{R}(\mathbf{x}) + \lambda \|\mathbf{R}_I \mathbf{x} - \mathbf{y}_I\|_p^p$, where $\mathcal{R}(\mathbf{x})$ is a regularizer and $\| \cdot \|_p$ denotes a norm which ensures data consistency. Typical choices for the regularizer are the total variation, or the ℓ^1-norm with respect to a frame or a trained dictionary. As a drawback, these methods are usually computationally expensive since they rely on a repeated application of the forward and adjoint operators. Furthermore, using regularization solely based on prior assumptions will likely bias the result.

Methods based on neural networks as for example in [4] propose non-iterative regularization approaches. Given an estimate solution $\mathbf{x}_I$ of (2), regularized images are obtained as the output of a CNN f which is previously trained on a dataset of pairs $(\mathbf{x}_I, \mathbf{x}_{\text{full}})$, where $\mathbf{x}_{\text{full}}$ is an image obtained from the reconstruction of a fully-sampled measurement. Such a procedure consists in a subsequent regularization of the initial solution $\mathbf{x}_I$ rather than a joint minimization of $\mathcal{R}(\mathbf{x}) + \lambda \|\mathbf{R}_I \mathbf{x} - \mathbf{y}_I\|_p^p$. Therefore, following [7], we propose to train different networks intercepted by data consistency (DC) layers.

2.1   Data Consistency Layer

Let f_Θ be a previously trained CNN with parameters Θ. Given measured data $\mathbf{y}_I$, we can apply a CNN to map $\mathbf{x}_I$ to its corresponding label, i.e. $f_\Theta(\mathbf{x}_I) \simeq \mathbf{x}_{\text{full}}$ where $\mathbf{x}_I \triangleq \mathbf{R}^\dagger \mathbf{y}_I$. However, the CNN reconstruction $f_\Theta(\mathbf{x}_I)$ may not satisfy the data consistency condition $\mathbf{R}_I(f_\Theta(\mathbf{x}_I)) \simeq \mathbf{y}_I$.

In order to improve data consistency, we define a new reconstruction $f_{\text{dc}}(\mathbf{x}_{\text{cnn}}, \mathbf{y}_I, \lambda) \triangleq \mathbf{R}^\dagger(\mathbf{z}_{\text{dc}})$ where $\mathbf{z}_{\text{dc}} \in \mathbb{R}^d$ is the minimizer of the functional given by

$$F_{\Theta, \mathbf{y}_I, \mathbf{x}_{\text{cnn}}, \lambda}(\mathbf{z}) \triangleq \|\mathbf{R}(\mathbf{x}_{\text{cnn}}) - \mathbf{z}\|_2^2 + \lambda \|\mathbf{y}_I - \mathbf{S}_I \mathbf{z}\|_2^2, \tag{3}$$

with $\mathbf{x}_{\text{cnn}} = f_\Theta(\mathbf{x}_I)$ denoting the output of the trained CNN.

Here, the term $\|\mathbf{y}_I - \mathbf{S}_I \mathbf{z}\|_2^2$ enforces data consistency and $\|\mathbf{R}(\mathbf{x}_{\text{cnn}}) - \mathbf{z}\|_2^2$ uses $\mathbf{x}_{\text{cnn}}$ to regularize in Radon space. Opposed to [7], where the regularization term $\|\mathbf{x}_{\text{cnn}} - \mathbf{x}\|_2^2$ in image space has been used, the proposed regularization in data space yields the following representation of the DC layer for general, possibly non-orthogonal transforms.

Theorem 1. *Let* $\mathbf{R} \in \mathbb{R}^{d \times n}$ *be a real valued matrix and* $\mathbf{R}_I = \mathbf{S}_I \mathbf{R}$, *where* $\mathbf{S}_I$ *is the subsampling operator defined in (1). The data consistency layer* $f_{\mathrm{dc}}(\mathbf{x}_{\mathrm{cnn}}, \mathbf{y}_I, \lambda)$ *is well defined by (3) and takes the explicit form*

$$f_{\mathrm{dc}}(\mathbf{x}_{\mathrm{cnn}}, \mathbf{y}_I, \lambda) = \mathbf{R}^\dagger \left(\mathbf{A} \mathbf{R} \mathbf{x}_{\mathrm{cnn}} + \frac{\lambda}{1+\lambda} \mathbf{y}_I \right), \tag{4}$$

where $\mathbf{A} = \mathrm{diag}(a_1, \ldots, a_n)$ *is a diagonal matrix of size* $d \times d$ *with diagonal entries* $a_i = 1$ *if* $i \notin I$ *and* $a_i = 1/(1+\lambda)$ *otherwise.*

Proof. The functional in (3) takes the separable form $\sum_{i \in J} |\mathbf{R} \mathbf{x}_{\mathrm{cnn}}(i) - \mathbf{z}(i)|_2^2 + \lambda |\mathbf{y}_I(i) - (\mathbf{S}_I \mathbf{z})(i)|_2^2$. Hence, the minimizer of $F_{\Theta, \mathbf{y}_I, \mathbf{x}_{\mathrm{cnn}}, \lambda}$ is unique and can be found by component-wise minimization. Elementary computations show (4). $\square$

The matrix $\mathbf{A}$ ensures that, when the i-th projection is not available from the measurements, $(\mathbf{R}\mathbf{x})(i)$ is directly estimated from the projection data of the output of the CNN. Otherwise, $(\mathbf{R}\mathbf{x})(i)$ is calculated as a linear combination of the CNN coefficient $\mathbf{R}\mathbf{x}_{\mathrm{cnn}}(i)$ and the measured coefficient $\mathbf{y}_I(i)$. Note that the evaluation of (4) requires the application of the pseudoinverse, which might be numerically unstable. In the numerical implementation, the pseudoinverse $\mathbf{R}^\dagger$ is replaced by an appropriate regularization. We emphasize that this issue is not present in MRI reconstruction, as the corresponding full data operator is bijective and the inverse well-conditioned. Therefore, the extension of the corresponding data consistency layer from MRI to CT is a non-trivial issue.

2.2   U-Nets Cascade

Here, we always refer to a U-net as any residual encoder-decoder network architecture with a similar structure to the one presented in [4]. However, in our experiments we vary the number of stages which are used to encode the input, the number of convolutional layers per stage, the initial number of feature maps which are extracted from the input and the factor by which the feature maps are augmented after each max-pooling layer. In order to satisfy the data consistency condition $\mathbf{R}_I(f_\Theta(\mathbf{x}_I)) \simeq \mathbf{y}_I$, we propose to construct a sequence of U-nets which are intercepted by DC layers as described in Subsect. 2.1. While the U-nets tackle the removal of the undersampling artifacts, the DC layers account for data consistency in Radon space. Figure 1 shows the structure of a U-nets cascade, where each U-net consists of three encoding stages and two convolutional layers per stage.

3   Numerical Experiments

3.1   Dataset

We test our proposed network architecture on a dataset consisting of cardiac CT images from 52 patients. The $3D$ volumes contain from 240 up to 640 slices per patient. For each slice, the undersampled data $\mathbf{y}_I$ is generated according to a

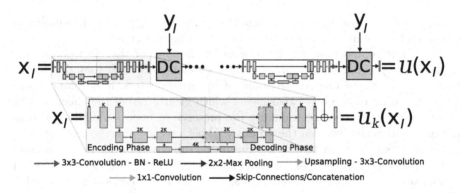

Fig. 1. A cascade of U-nets with intermediate data consistency layers.

parallel-beam geometry where we cover a half rotation of 180° of the scanner by only 32 angles. The images $\mathbf{x}_I$ are obtained by applying filtered back-projection $\mathbf{R}^\dagger$ with Ram-Lak filter to $\mathbf{y}_I$. The operator $\mathbf{R}$ is assumed to perform 512 projections. We use the images of 40 patients for training, of 6 for validation and of 6 for testing. For computational reasons and in order to allow us to build neural networks with a certain depth, the images are first downsampled from 512×512 to 256×256 pixels.

3.2 Network Architectures and Training

In all our experiments we train the U-nets cascade to minimize the L_2-error between the predicted output of the cascade and the corresponding label. All architectures are trained for 20 epochs by stochastic gradient descent. When one single U-net is used, we decrease the learning rate from 10^{-7} to 10^{-9}. For all other architectures which contain the operators $\mathbf{R}$ and $\mathbf{R}^\dagger$, a more conservative learning rate which is decreased from 10^{-10} to 10^{-14} has to be chosen for numerical stability. The network architectures are implemented in `TensorFlow` and the scanner geometry, the forward and the pseudoinverse operators $\mathbf{R}$ and $\mathbf{R}^\dagger$ are implemented in `ODL` [1]. We parametrize a U-net cascade according to the following hyperparameters:

- U - the number of U-nets employed in the cascade
- E - the number of stages used for the encoding of each U-net
- C - the number of convolutional layers per stage for each U-net
- K - the number of feature maps which are initially extracted from the input of each U-net
- F - the factor by which the number of feature maps is increased after the max-pooling layers of each U-net.

For example, U1 E5 C4 K64 F2 denotes a single U-net architecture similar to the one presented in [4]. On the other hand, U4 E1 C4 K64 denotes a FCNN cascade as discussed in [7]. Note that, in such a case, we omit the hyperparameter F in the notation, since due to the absence of max-pooling layers, the number of extracted feature maps stays constant over the different stages.

For a fair comparison, we try to keep the number of trainable parameters approximately equal for the architectures we compare. Note that due to the large number of possible combinations of hyperparameters, it is computationally demanding to conduct experiments which clearly reveal the effect of each hyperparamter. However, we identify the presence of max-pooling layers to be the main difference between the proposed U-net cascade and the cascade in [7] in terms of feature-extraction-operations of the subnetworks. Therefore, in order to reach a certain number of trainable parameters, we choose to always favour to increase the number of encoding stages rather than increasing the number of convolutional layers per stage, the number of extracted feature maps or the factor by which they are increased after the max-pooling layers.

For the evaluation of the performance of the network we report the peak signal-to-noise ratio (PSNR), the relative L_2-error (NRMSE), the structural similarity index measure (SSIM) and the Haar-wavelet based perceptual similarity index measure (HPSI, [5]) which has been reported to achieve higher correlation with human opinion scores than SSIM on various benchmark databases.

Effect of the U-Net: Here, we investigate the effect of the replacement of the FCNNs discussed in [7] by the U-nets. Table 1 lists the average of the aforementioned quantitative measures over the test set. In terms of PSNR, SSIM and NRMSE, both cascades deliver similar results. On the other hand, we report a statistically significant increase of the mean value of HPSI for all tested U-nets cascades, ($p < 0.001$ for all cases). Figure 2 shows two examples of reconstructed images of the test set. Due the relatively small number of trainable parameters and the high undersampling factor, both approaches do not entirely remove the

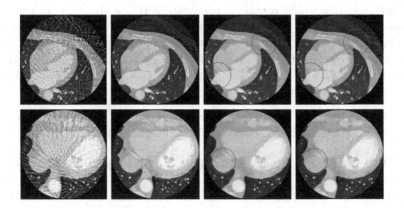

Fig. 2. Comparison of different cascades. 32-views FBP-reconstruction (first column), ground truth (second column), U4 E1 C4 K64 (third column), U4 E4 C2 K32 (fourth column). The red circles indicate newly introduced or not correctly removed artifacts from the reconstruction with the FCNNs-cascade. (Color figure online)

undersampling artifacts and fail at recovering fine details. Note that, however, the cascade with the FCNNs even introduces new artifacts. The phenomenon can be observed in several images reconstructed with the FCNNs cascade. On the other hand, the U-nets cascade seems to better preserve the overall structure of the images.

Table 1. Comparison of the proposed U-nets cascade with a cascade of FCNNs with residual connections. The measures are averaged over the test set.

Model	n_{params}	PSNR	SSIM	HPSI	NRMSE
U2 E1 C4 K64	371 459	30.63	0.8961	0.7236	0.1597
U2 E4 C2 K32	352 899	30.56	0.8939	0.7433	0.1612
U3 E1 C4 K64	557 187	30.26	0.8737	0.7311	0.1692
U3 E4 C2 K32	529 347	30.33	0.8744	0.7499	0.1679
U4 E1 C4 K64	742 915	29.89	0.8581	0.7326	0.1799
U4 E4 C2 K32	705 795	29.92	0.8603	0.7540	0.1782

Effect of the Cascade: In this experiment, we test different network architectures where we vary the length of the cascade. Figure 3 shows an image reconstructed with different network cascades. The results show that the left coronary artery is better visible in the images reconstructed with the U-nets cascades compared to a single U-net. In contrast to the results presented in [7], increasing the

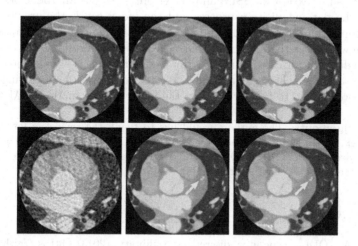

Fig. 3. Variation of the length of the cascade. Ground truth (top left), FBP-reconstruction from undersampled data (bottom left), U1 E3 C2 K64 F2-reconstruction (top middle), U2 E3 C4 K32 F2-reconstruction (bottom middle), U3 E3 C3 K64-reconstruction (top right), U4 E3 C2 K32 F2-reconstruction (bottom right). The yellow arrows point at the left coronary artery. (Color figure online)

Table 2. Variation of the length of the U-nets cascade. The measures are averaged over the test set.

Model	n_{params}	PSNR	SSIM	HPSI	NRMSE
U1 E3 C2 K64 F2	1 957 251	30.19	0.9532	0.7304	0.1832
U2 E3 C4 K32 F2	1 941 379	31.14	0.8905	0.7659	0.1531
U3 E3 C3 K64	1 999 107	30.85	0.8686	0.7732	0.1621
U4 E3 C2 K32 F2	1 960 707	30.38	0.8559	0.7729	0.1732

length of the cascades does not further improve the results. We attribute this to the fact that the inversion of the Radon-transform is ill-posed and therefore, numerical errors due to the inversion of $\mathbf{R}$ prevail over the presence of the data consistency layers. However, when we replace a single U-net by a U-nets cascade, the network's performance statistically significantly increases ($p < 0.001$) with respect to all measures except for SSIM, where a single U-net yields the best results, see Table 2.

3.3   Conclusion

In this work, we have presented a new network architecture for image reconstruction in sparse view CT. Replacing the FCNNs by U-nets in the cascade in [7] visually improves the reconstruction in sparse view CT. The proposed U-nets cascade outperforms the single U-net architecture with respect to all reported quantitative measures except for SSIM and better preserves fine anatomic details. By adapting the data-acquisition process and the index set I, the architecture is directly applicable to other limited data inverse problems such as limited angle CT where we expect the method to deliver even better results as the portion of measured data which can be used in the reconstruction is significantly larger. Furthermore, we expect the extension of the network cascade employing U-nets as sub-networks also to further improve the image reconstruction in MRI.

Acknowledgements. The authors would like to thank the reviewers for the helpful feedback. A. Kofler acknowledges support of the German Research Foundation (DFG), project number GRK 2260, BIOQIC. M. Haltmeier acknowledges support of the Austrian Science Fund (FWF), project P 30747-N32.

References

1. Jonas, A.: ODL - operator discretization library (2013). https://github.com/odlgroup/odl
2. Adler, J., Öktem, O.: Solving ill-posed inverse problems using iterative deep neural networks. Inverse Prob. **33**(12), 124007 (2017)
3. Hammernik, K., et al.: Learning a variational network for reconstruction of accelerated MRI data. Magn. Reson. Med. **79**(6), 3055–3071 (2018)

4. Jin, K.H., McCann, M.T., Froustey, E., Unser, M.: Deep convolutional neural network for inverse problems in imaging. IEEE Trans. Image Process. **26**(9), 4509–4522 (2017)
5. Reisenhofer, R., Bosse, S., Kutyniok, G., Wiegand, T.: A Haar wavelet-based perceptual similarity index for image quality assessment. Signal Process. Image Commun. **61**, 33–43 (2018)
6. Ronneberger, O., Fischer, P., Brox, T.: U-Net: convolutional networks for biomedical image segmentation. In: Navab, N., Hornegger, J., Wells, W.M., Frangi, A.F. (eds.) MICCAI 2015. LNCS, vol. 9351, pp. 234–241. Springer, Cham (2015). https://doi.org/10.1007/978-3-319-24574-4_28
7. Schlemper, J., Caballero, J., Hajnal, J.V., Price, A., Rueckert, D.: A deep cascade of convolutional neural networks for MR image reconstruction. In: Niethammer, M. (ed.) IPMI 2017. LNCS, vol. 10265, pp. 647–658. Springer, Cham (2017). https://doi.org/10.1007/978-3-319-59050-9_51

Deep Learning for General Image Reconstruction

Approximate k-Space Models and Deep Learning for Fast Photoacoustic Reconstruction

Andreas Hauptmann[1]([✉]), Ben Cox[2], Felix Lucka[1,3], Nam Huynh[2],
Marta Betcke[1], Paul Beard[2], and Simon Arridge[1]

[1] Department of Computer Science, University College London, London, UK
a.hauptmann@ucl.ac.uk
[2] Department of Medical Physics and Biomedical Engineering,
University College London, London, UK
[3] Centrum Wiskunde & Informatica, Amsterdam, Netherlands

Abstract. We present a framework for accelerated iterative reconstructions using a fast and approximate forward model that is based on k-space methods for photoacoustic tomography. The approximate model introduces aliasing artefacts in the gradient information for the iterative reconstruction, but these artefacts are highly structured and we can train a CNN that can use the approximate information to perform an iterative reconstruction. We show feasibility of the method for human in-vivo measurements in a limited-view geometry. The proposed method is able to produce superior results to total variation reconstructions with a speed-up of 32 times.

Keywords: Learned image reconstruction
Photoacoustic tomography · Fast fourier methods · Compressed sensing

1 Introduction

There is increasing interest in Photoacoustic tomography (PAT) for both clinical and preclinical imaging [1], as it has the potential to provide molecular and functional information with high spatial resolution [2]. For preclinical imaging it is often possible to make measurements all around the object, but for clinical imaging, PAT scanners with access to just one side of the tissue are typically required. In addition, clinical imaging typically requires high frame rates [3]. The frame rate is determined both by the time taken for the data acquisition as well as by the image reconstruction time. Compressed sensing can dramatically reduce data acquisition time, but then suitable image reconstruction approaches are required, which are typically slow due to the large number of iterations required. This paper proposes to use an approximate and fast model within a deep learning framework for PAT image reconstruction from sparse data measured using a planar scanner.

© Springer Nature Switzerland AG 2018
F. Knoll et al. (Eds.): MLMIR 2018, LNCS 11074, pp. 103–111, 2018.
https://doi.org/10.1007/978-3-030-00129-2_12

2   Forward and Inverse Models

2.1   Photoacoustic Tomography

In PAT, a short pulse of near-infrared light is absorbed by chromophores in tissue. For a sufficiently short pulse, a spatially-varying pressure increase f will result, which will initiate an ultrasound (US) pulse (*photoacoustic effect*), which then propagates to the tissue surface. The measurement consists of the detected waves in space-time at the boundary of the tissue; this set of pressure time series constitutes the PA data g. This acoustic propagation is commonly modeled by the following initial value problem for the wave equation [4],

$$(\partial_{tt} - c^2 \Delta)p(\mathbf{x}, t) = 0, \quad p(\mathbf{x}, t = 0) = f(\mathbf{x}), \quad \partial_t p(\mathbf{x}, t = 0) = 0. \tag{1}$$

The measurement of the PA signal is then modeled as a linear operator $\mathcal{M}$ acting on the pressure field $p(\mathbf{x}, t)$ restricted to the boundary of the computational domain Ω and a finite time window (see [2,5] for details on measurement systems):

$$g = \mathcal{M} p_{|\partial\Omega \times (0,T)}. \tag{2}$$

Equations (1) and (2) define a linear mapping

$$Af = g, \tag{3}$$

from initial pressure f to measured pressure time series g, which constitutes the acoustic *forward problem* in PAT. The corresponding image reconstruction step constitutes the acoustic *inverse problem* to (3).

2.2   Fast Approximate Forward and Inverse Models

When the measurement points lie on a plane ($z = 0$) outside the support of f, the pressure there can be related to f by [4]:

$$p(x, y, t) = \frac{1}{c^2} \mathcal{F}_{k_x, k_y} \left\{ \left\{ \mathcal{C}_\omega \left\{ B(k_x, k_y, \omega) \tilde{f}(k_x, k_y, \omega) \right\} \right\} \right\}, \tag{4}$$

where $\tilde{f}(k_x, k_y, \omega)$ is obtained from $\hat{f}(\mathbf{k})$ via the dispersion relation $(\omega/c)^2 = k_x^2 + k_y^2 + k_z^2$ and $\hat{f}(\mathbf{k}) = \mathcal{F}_\mathbf{x}\{f(\mathbf{x})\}$ is the 3D Fourier transform of $f(\mathbf{x})$. $\mathcal{C}_\omega$ is a cosine transform from ω to t, $\mathcal{F}_{k_x, k_y}$ is the 2D inverse Fourier Transform on the detector plane. The weighting factor,

$$B(k_x, k_y, \omega) = \omega / \left(\mathrm{sgn}(\omega) \sqrt{(\omega/c)^2 - k_x^2 - k_y^2} \right), \tag{5}$$

contains an integrable singularity which means that if Eq. (4) is evaluated by discretisation on a rectangular grid, (thus enabling the application of FFT for efficient calculation), then aliasing in $p(x, y, t)$ results. An accurate model employing Eq. (4) would require suitable measures to deal with the singularity, whereas evaluation using FFT leads to a *fast but approximate* forward model. To control the degree of aliasing, all components of B for which $k_x^2 + k_y^2 > (\omega/c)^2 \sin^2 \theta_{max}$ were set to zero. This is equivalent to assuming only waves arriving at angles up to θ_{max} from normal incidence are detected. There is a trade-off: the greater the range of angles included, the greater the aliasing, as illustrated in Fig. 1.

By inverting Eq. 4, it can also be used as a method for mapping from the measured data g to an estimate of f [6]. In this case, there is no singularity to contend with, but the estimate of f will suffer from limited-view artifacts [7]. We will denote these two k-space methods as $A_{\mathcal{F}}$ and $A_{\mathcal{F}}^\dagger$ for the forward and backward projections, respectively.

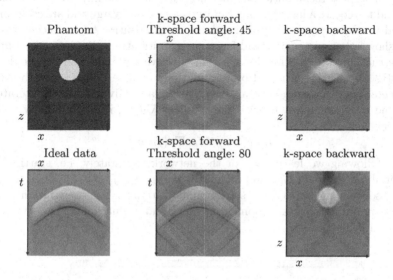

Fig. 1. Approximate forward model. Top left: 2D phantom with a line detector (red line). Bottom left: ideal data. The effect of two different levels of angle thresholding of the incident waves is shown in the middle column and the resulting backprojection of the approximate data in the right column. (Color figure online)

3   Learned Reconstruction with Approximate Models

In order to use an approximate forward model, such as described above, in an iterative reconstruction method, a correction must be incorporated. Here Deep Learning, specifically convolutional neural networks, offer an ideal framework to learn a correction to an approximate model. This can be done in two ways, either by learning an explicit correction of the forward model and subsequently applying an iterative scheme, or learning the correction inside a learned iterative reconstruction scheme. This study will concentrate on the second approach.

3.1 Learned Iterative Reconstruction

Photoacoustic reconstructions from subsampled data measured over a limited detection aperture are typically computed by solving a variational problem as the minimisation of the sum of a data-fidelity term and a regularisation, $\mathcal{R}$, term enforcing certain regularities of the solution f^* as

$$f^* = \arg\min_f \frac{1}{2}\|Af - g\|_2^2 + \alpha\mathcal{R}(f), \tag{6}$$

where $\alpha > 0$ is a weighting parameter. It has been shown in several studies [8–11] that these techniques can efficiently deal with the limited view artefacts, but tend to require a larger number of iterations to converge and are additionally limited by the expressibility of the chosen regularisation term. Recently it has been shown that one can instead learn such an iterative scheme to speed up the reconstruction and additionally learn an effective regularisation for the data at hand [12–14]. This is achieved by formulating a simple CNN G_{θ_k}, with learned parameters θ_k, that computes an iterative update. Given a current iterate f_k, then the CNN combines f_k with the gradient $\nabla d(f_k, g)$ of the fidelity term in (6), such that

$$f_{k+1} = G_{\theta_k}(f_k, \nabla d(f_k, g)). \tag{7}$$

In the following we learn each of the networks separately; i.e. starting with an initial f_0, we train G_{θ_0} and compute the update f_1 by (7). Then we train the subsequent networks for a set amount of iterates. This separation is done due to computational restrictions in memory and evaluation of the forward and backward projections.

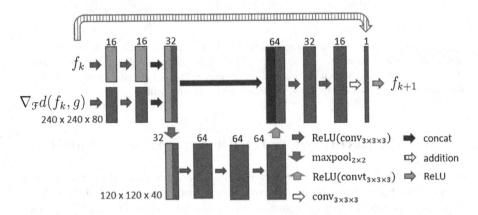

Fig. 2. Network architecture for an iterative gradient update with approximate models. Each network gets the iterate f_k and the approximate gradient information $\nabla_{\mathcal{F}} d(f_k, g) := A_{\mathcal{F}}^\dagger(A_{\mathcal{F}} f_k - g)$ as input. The output f_{k+1} is a residual update to the previous iterate. The multiscale structure is introduced to remove artefacts from the gradient.

3.2   An Iterative Gradient Network

We propose to use an approximate model $A_{\mathcal{F}}$ as described in Sect. 2.2. This model will be used to compute the gradient information in (7), i.e. we have $\nabla_{\mathcal{F}} d(f_k, g) := A_{\mathcal{F}}^\dagger (A_{\mathcal{F}} f_k - g) \approx \nabla d(f_k, g)$. By the application of the fast and approximate forward model we introduce artefacts to the gradient information, but these are highly structured, as illustrated in Fig. 1. Multiscale networks, such as a residual U-Net, have been proven to be efficient in detecting and removing artefacts in images [15]. Thus, we believe that a multiscale network can be efficiently used to remove these artefacts. On the other hand, smaller gradient informed networks are more robust to perturbations in the measurement geometry or the imaged target, as suggested in [14].

In this work we propose to balance both approaches, by combining a deep gradient descent network proposed in [14] with a small mutliscale network in order to deal successfully with artefacts in the gradient, while still possessing the ability to generalise well with respect to changes in the measurement geometry. The particular network structure chosen for this application is illustrated in Fig. 2. The two inputs, current iterate f_k and the approximate gradient $\nabla_{\mathcal{F}} d(f_k, g)$, go through two separate convolutional pipelines with filter size 3^3. The results are then combined by concatenation and downsampled with a maxpool layer to a courser scale. The result of the courser scale is concatenated with the result of the two initial convolutional pipelines and the channel size successively reduced to one channel, which is added as a residual update to the input iterate f_k and projected onto the positive set to produce the new iterate f_{k+1}.

4   Computational Results for In-Vivo Measurements

4.1   Data Acquisition and Preparation

In-vivo measurements of a human subject have been taken with the planar sensor described in [16]. For faster acquisition the scanner uses a 16 beam interrogation laser to measure the PA signal. In total we obtained 27 fully-sampled limited-view measurements used in this study. Since this is not sufficient for training an iterative reconstruction algorithm, we have additionally used a large dataset of 1024 volumes of blood vessels segmented from lung CT scans as described in [14] of size $240 \times 240 \times 80$. We then simulated accurate sub-sampled limited-view photoacoustic measurement data of the segmented lung vessels with a sub-sampling factor of 4 and a randomly generated 16 beam sub-sampling pattern for each sample, (see Fig. 3 for example patterns). Additionally, we have varied the sound speed in the simulations to be uniformly distributed in $[1560\text{m/s}, 1600\text{m/s}]$ and added normally distributed noise to the data with varying intensity, such that the resulting signal's SNR is roughly between 10 to 30. These variations have been done to increase robustness to variations in the measurements.

16 beam scanner sampling pattern

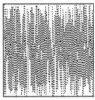

Fig. 3. Randomly generated sub-sampling pattern with the 16 beam scanner geometry and a sub-sampling factor of 4; black dots indicate interrogated points on the sensor. (Left) Pattern used for experimental sample I, (Right) pattern used for experimental sample II.

4.2   Training of Proposed Network

We have pre-trained the networks G_{θ_k} on the simulated data from segmented lung vessels. Given the simulated measurement g, the initial reconstruction is computed by the k-space backprojection, i.e. $f_0 = A_{\mathcal{F}}^{\dagger} g$, as described in Sect. 2.2. We have trained in total 5 iterative networks G_{θ_k} for $k = 0, \ldots, 4$. Each network is trained in TensorFlow with the Adam algorithm for 30 epochs with an initial learning rate of $2 \cdot 10^{-4}$ and a ℓ^2-loss. The training of each iterate takes about 14 hours; with initialisation and computations between iterates the whole pre-training takes a bit under 4 days on a single Titan Xp GPU.

After pre-training we have taken 25 of the in-vivo measurements and produced synthetically 4 times sub-sampled data with a 16 beam pattern. As reference reconstruction we have taken a total variation (TV) constrained reconstruction of the fully-sampled limited-view data. We have then performed an update training of the pre-trained networks with the 25 samples to adjust the algorithm to in-vivo artefacts not present in simulated data. The update training is performed for 8 epochs with a learning rate of 10^{-4} and we minimised the ℓ^2-error to the reference TV reconstructions from fully-sampled limited-view data.

4.3   Reconstructions of In-Vivo Measurements

The reconstruction with the trained network is performed on 2 samples of in-vivo limited-view measurements with 4 times sub-sampling, the corresponding sub-sampling pattern is shown in Fig. 3. The resulting reconstructions for both samples are shown in Figs. 4 and 5. Evaluation of the projections take each 1.6 s and of the network 0.45 s, hence one iterate takes a bit less than 4 s. The total computation time for 5 iterates with initialisation is about 20 s on a single Titan Xp GPU. For comparison we have computed TV reconstructions of the same sub-sampled data for both test cases. The regularisation parameter was chosen, such that PSNR to the reference reconstruction is maximised. The resulting reconstructions are shown in Fig. 6 and take approximately 11 min.

Initial backprojection   FF-PAT, 5 iterations   fully-sampled reference

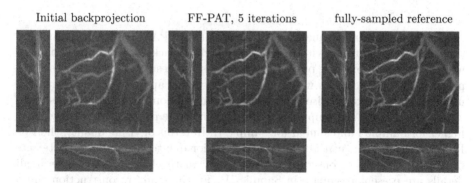

Fig. 4. Sample I: reconstruction of in-vivo measurements from 4× undersampled 16-beam pattern (maximum intensity projections). PSNR in comparison to the reference from fully-sampled limited-view data: backprojection 33.5672, FF-PAT 42.1749.

Initial backprojection   FF-PAT, 5 iterations   fully-sampled reference

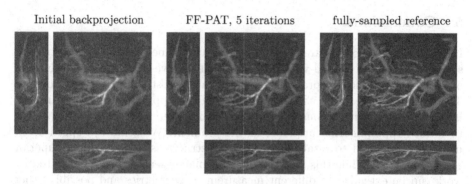

Fig. 5. Sample II: reconstruction of in-vivo measurements from 4× undersampled 16 beam pattern (maximum intensity projections). PSNR in comparison to the reference from fully-sampled limited-view data: backprojection 34.4372, FF-PAT 42.0388.

Sample I   Sample II

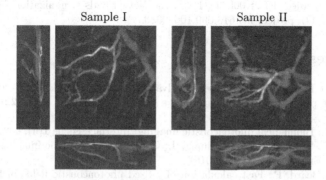

Fig. 6. TV reconstructions (20 iterations, maximum intensity projections) of in-vivo measurements from 4× undersampled 16-beam pattern. PSNR in comparison to the reference from fully-sampled limited-view data: Sample I 41.1576, Sample II 42.1391.

4.4   Discussion

In both cases, the image quality of the Fast Forward PAT (FF-PAT) reconstructions is clearly improved with respect to the initial backprojection. Even though we have used approximate projection operators, the results suggest that the proposed network generalises well and incorporates the approximate gradient in a useful manner. In comparison to the TV reconstruction, FF-PAT is competitive with respect to PSNR computed in comparison to the reference reconstructions: higher for Sample I and similar for Sample II. In terms of visual quality, the FF-PAT reconstructions can be considered superior due to strong blocky artefacts present in the TV reconstructions, especially in the background where small details are present (compare in Sample II). Furthermore, reconstruction times are reduced by a factor of 32. In comparison to learned iterative reconstructions with the accurate model, see [14], image quality is competitive with a speed-up of FF-PAT by factor 8.

5   Conclusions

Iterative reconstructions are necessary in restricted measurement geometries to successively negate limited-view artefacts. This involves the repeated evaluation of forward and backward projections, which can be costly in high-resolution and 3D. We have successfully shown that one can use approximate models instead in a learned iterative reconstruction algorithm, where the network also learns to negate approximation artefacts in the gradient. We achieve a speed-up of up to 32 compared to established TV reconstructions and providing superior reconstructions. While this study applies for planar sensors in PAT, the framework can be extended to different measurement geometries and possibly other modalities.

Acknowledgment. Support of NVIDIA Corporation with one Titan Xp GPU. AH is supported from the Wellcome-EPSRC project NS/A000027/1. FL is supported from EPSRC project EP/K009745/1 and the Netherlands Organization for Scientific Research (NWO), project nr. 613.009.106/2383.

References

1. Upputuri, P., Pramanik, M.: Recent advances toward preclinical and clinical translation of photoacoustic tomography: a review. J. Biomed. Opt. **22**(4), 041006 (2016)
2. Beard, P.: Biomedical photoacoustic imaging. Interface Focus **1**(4), 602–631 (2011)
3. Choi, W., Seungwan, E., Chulhong, J.: Clinical photoacoustic imaging platforms. Biomed. Eng. Lett. **7**, 1–17 (2018)
4. Cox, B., Beard, P.: Fast calculation of pulsed photoacoustic fields in fluids using k-space methods. J. Acoust. Soc. Am. **117**(6), 3616–3627 (2005)
5. Lutzweiler, C., Razansky, D.: Optoacoustic imaging and tomography: reconstruction approaches and outstanding challenges in image performance and quantification. Sensors **13**(6), 7345 (2013)

6. Köstli, K., Frenz, M., Bebie, H., Weber, H.: Temporal backward projection of optoacoustic pressure transients using Fourier transform methods. Phys. Med. Biol. **46**(7), 1863–1872 (2001)
7. Xu, Y., Wang, L., Ambartsoumian, G., Kuchment, P.: Reconstructions in limited-view thermoacoustic tomography. Med. Phys. **31**(4), 724–733 (2004)
8. Huang, C., Wang, K., Nie, L., Wang, L.V., Anastasio, M.: Full-wave iterative image reconstruction in photoacoustic tomography with acoustically inhomogeneous media. IEEE Trans. Med. Imaging **32**(6), 1097–1110 (2013)
9. Arridge, S., Betcke, M., Cox, B., Lucka, F., Treeby, B.: On the adjoint operator in photoacoustic tomography. Inverse Probl. **32**(11), 115012 (2016)
10. Arridge, S.R., et al.: Accelerated high-resolution photoacoustic tomography via compressed sensing. Phys. Med. Biol. **61**(24), 8908 (2016)
11. Boink, Y.E., Lagerwerf, M.J., Steenbergen, W., van Gils, S.A., Manohar, S., Brune, C.: A framework for directional and higher-order reconstruction in photoacoustic tomography. Phys. Med. Biol. **63**(4), 045018 (2018)
12. Hammernik, K., et al.: Learning a variational network for reconstruction of accelerated MRI data. Magn. Reson. Med. **79**(6), 3055–3071 (2018)
13. Adler, J., Öktem, O.: Solving ill-posed inverse problems using iterative deep neural networks. Inverse Probl. **33**(12), 124007 (2017)
14. Hauptmann, M., et al.: Model based learning for accelerated, limited-view 3D photoacoustic tomography. IEEE Trans. Med. Imag. **37**(6), 1382–1393 (2018)
15. Jin, K., McCann, M., Froustey, E., Unser, M.: Deep convolutional neural network for inverse problems in imaging. IEEE Trans. Image Process. **26**(9), 4509–4522 (2017)
16. Huynh, N., Ogunlade, O., Zhang, E., Cox, B., Beard, P.: Photoacoustic imaging using an 8-beam Fabry-perot scanner. In: Photons Plus Ultrasound: Imaging and Sensing 2016, vol. 9708, p. 97082L (2016)

Deep Learning Based Image Reconstruction for Diffuse Optical Tomography

Hanene Ben Yedder[1(✉)], Aïcha BenTaieb[1], Majid Shokoufi[2],
Amir Zahiremami[2], Farid Golnaraghi[2], and Ghassan Hamarneh[1]

[1] School of Computing Science, Simon Fraser University, Burnaby, Canada
{hbenyedd,abentaie,hamarneh}@sfu.ca
[2] School of Mechatronic Systems Engineering, Simon Fraser University,
Surrey, Canada
{mshokouf,azahirem,mfgolnar}@sfu.ca

Abstract. Diffuse optical tomography (DOT) is a relatively new imaging modality that has demonstrated its clinical potential of probing tumors in a non-invasive and affordable way. Image reconstruction is an ill-posed challenging task because knowledge of the exact analytic inverse transform does not exist a priori, especially in the presence of sensor non-idealities and noise. Standard reconstruction approaches involve approximating the inverse function and often require expert parameters tuning to optimize reconstruction performance. In this work, we evaluate the use of a deep learning model to reconstruct images directly from their corresponding DOT projection data. The inverse problem is solved by training the model via training pairs created using physics-based simulation. Both quantitative and qualitative results indicate the superiority of the proposed network compared to an analytic technique.

Keywords: Diffuse optical tomography · Inverse problem
Reconstruction · Deep learning

1 Introduction

Breast cancer, the most common cancer among women, is ranked as the second leading cause of cancer-related death, in North America. Annually, 1.3 million new cases of breast cancer are diagnosed worldwide [1]. Prescreening is typically carried out using clinical breast examination or self-breast examinations that suffers from high false-positive rates. Ultrasound, X-ray mammography, and magnetic resonance imaging (MRI) are the most commonly used imaging modalities for breast cancer detection. While X-ray mammography is the primary screening technique, it is often a painful exam that is mainly recommended for women over the age of 50, due to its low sensitivity (67.8%) for younger women or women with dense breasts as well as its potential health risk due to its ionizing

© Springer Nature Switzerland AG 2018
F. Knoll et al. (Eds.): MLMIR 2018, LNCS 11074, pp. 112–119, 2018.
https://doi.org/10.1007/978-3-030-00129-2_13

radiation. Ultrasound and MRI modalities are well adapted for differentiating benign and malignant masses in dense breast tissue, however, ultrasound suffers from higher false positive rates compared to mammography and its effectiveness varies depending on the skill of the technician, whereas MRI is more costly and associated with long wait times [2].

New research [3,4] focuses on a novel imaging modality for breast cancer based on near-infrared (NIR) diffuse optical tomography (DOT), a non-invasive and non-ionising imaging modality that has demonstrated its clinical potential in probing tumors. DOT is a particularly-beneficial diagnostic method for women with dense breast tissue. DOT enables measuring and visualizing the distribution of tissue absorption and scattering properties where these optical parameters are related to physiological markers, e.g., blood oxygenation and tissue metabolism. When multiple wavelengths are used, DOT can map deoxyhemoglobin and oxy-hemoglobin concentrations, which in turn can be used to quantitatively assess tissue malignancy from total hemoglobin concentration.

Recently, we developed a new functional hand-held diffuse optical breast scanner probe (DOB-Scan) [5] that has been applied to breast cancer detection as a screening tool and aims to improve the assessment parameters in terms of positive predictive value and accuracy. The probe is currently in clinical trials for in vivo breast cancer imaging studies. It combines multi-frequency and continuous-wave near-infrared light to quantify tissue optical properties in 690 to 850 nm spectra and produces a cross-sectional image of the underneath tissue. The proposed probe uses encapsulated light emitting diodes instead of laser-coupled fiber-optic, which decreases the complexity, size, and cost of the probe while providing accurate and reliable optical properties measurement of the tissue. In this work, we focus on improving the image reconstruction from DOB-Scan probe measurements using machine learning technique.

Image reconstruction methods are mostly analytic and often suffer from well-known reconstruction problems, e.g., noise, motion artifacts, image degradation due to short acquisition time, and computational complexity [6]. Iterative reconstruction algorithms have become the dominant approach for solving inverse problems over the past few decades [7]. While iterative reconstruction with regularization, e.g., total variation, provides a way to mitigate some of the shortcomings of analytic reconstruction it remains difficult to obtain a method that is fast, provides high-resolution images, and requires a simple calibration process [8].

A more recent trend is machine learning based image reconstruction, which is motivated by the outstanding performance of deep learning on computer vision problems tasks, e.g., object classification and segmentation. Convolutional neural networks (CNNs) have previously been applied to medical image reconstruction problems in computed tomography and MRI [9–11]. Many approaches [6,12,13] obtain an initial estimate of the reconstruction using a direct inverse operator or an iterative approach, then use machine learning to refine the estimate and produce the final reconstructed image. Although this is a straightforward solution, the number of iterations required to obtain a reasonable initial image estimate can be hard to define and in general increases the total reconstruction run-time.

A more elegant solution is to reconstruct an image from its equivalent projection data directly by learning all the parameters of a deep neural network, in an end-to-end fashion and therefore, approximates the underlying physics of the inverse problem. In [14], a unified framework for image reconstruction that allows a mapping between sensor and image domain is proposed. A pre-trained CNN model is used to learn a bidirectional mapping between sensor and image domains where image reconstruction is formulated in a manifold learning framework. The trained model is tested on a variety of MRI acquisition strategies.

While deep learning based image reconstruction has been applied to a variety of medical imaging modalities, they have not yet been used for DOT. In this paper, we propose a deep DOT reconstruction method to learn a mapping between raw acquired measurements and reconstructed images. The raw collected data can be considered as image features that approximate nonlinear combinations of image pixel values, which form the desired tissue optical coefficients. Therefore, the raw measured data is a nonlinear function of the desired image pixels values and so performing image reconstruction amounts to learning to invert this nonlinear function. We propose to use deep neural networks to learn, from training data, this nonlinear inverse mapping.

To train our model, we rely on synthetic datasets of image pairs and their corresponding measurements that simulate real-world DOT signals. We leverage a physics-based optical diffusion simulator to generate these synthetic datasets. We evaluate our system on real measurements on phantom datasets collected with the NIR DOB-Scan probe and show the utility of our synthetic data generation technique in mimicking real measurements and the generalization ability of our model to unseen phantom datasets. The performance of our proposed system shows that our framework improves reconstruction accuracy when compared against a baseline analytic reconstruction approach.

2   Methodology

Our main goal is to reconstruct tomographic images from corresponding sensor-domain sampled data or measurements. To this end we collect training measurements from (a) synthesized tissue geometries with known optical properties using a physics-based simulation of the forward projection operation, and (b) data collected using the probe on physical phantoms. We describe the generation of synthetic training datasets as well as the design of the neural network architecture below.

2.1   Generating Training Data for DOT Reconstruction

Synthetic Datasets: Our aim here is to create training data pairs in-silico, which include image of optical tissue property and its corresponding measurement. The deep learning model will then be trained to generate the image from the measurement. We synthesize different geometries of tissue, i.e. different breast shapes and sizes and different lesion shapes, sizes, and locations, and model them as 2D triangular meshes. We then assign to these geometries optical transport parameters (absorption and scattering coefficients) similar to real human breast tissue and lesion distribution values [15].

To collect synthetic DOT measurements, we used the Toast++ software suite [16], which simulates the forward projection operation to generate projection measurements for each training mesh. Modelling the probe sources and detectors accurately in Toast++ was a critical step in obtaining realistic measurements that mimic real values obtained by the DOT probe. The source model we created consisted of two light sources that deliver near-infrared light to a body surface at different points. The detector model is defined as a row of detectors that measure the back-scattered light from the tissue and emitted from the boundary. The simulated light source and detectors' spatial distribution were defined to mimic the probe geometry detailed in [5], which comprise 2 LED light sources that illuminate tissue symmetrically and surround 128 detectors. Both LED and all detectors are colinear as depicted in Fig. 1. The forward projection simulation captures a 1D raw intensity diffraction resulting from the scattering of the illuminating light exiting the test object.

Phantom Dataset: To create physical phantom datasets we rely on a tissue-equivalent solution where an intralipid solution is used to mimic background breast tissue due to its similarity in optical properties to breast fat [3,4]. Measurements are collected with the DOB-Scan probe. In order to mimic cancerous lesions, a tube with 4 mm cross-sectional diameter was filled with a tumor-like liquid phantom (Indian black ink solution) and was placed at different locations inside the intralipid solution container. The flowchart of synthetic and phantom data acquisition procedures are shown in Fig. 2 (Left side).

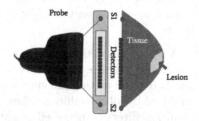

Fig. 1. The spatial distribution of the simulated sources and detectors matching the layout of the physical probe (left). A sample synthetic mesh is also shown (right).

2.2   Reconstructing Images from DOT Measurements

By passing an input measurement through a set of nonlinear transformations one can reconstruct the equivalent image. The proposed architecture consists of a dense layer followed by a set of convolution layers which are designed to efficiently combine features from the first layer with those of deeper layers. The architecture of our proposed model is shown in Fig. 2 (right side).

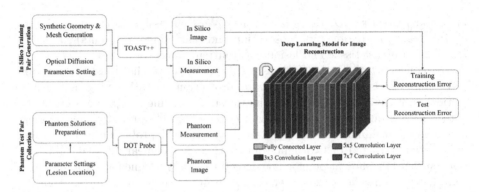

Fig. 2. In silico training pairs generation using TOAST++ and phantom test pairs collection using DOT-probe are depicted on the left. The overall architecture of the proposed model is shown on the right, where the arrow after the first fully connected layer represents the reshaping procedure before the convolution layers.

Initial Image Estimate: A fully connected layer, with a ReLu activation, is used as the first layer of the network in order to map the measurement vector to a two-dimensional array that will serve as an initial image estimate. This layer is first pre-trained then included in the deeper architecture including convolutional layers. The goal we seek to achieve using the fully connected layer is to generalize the filtered back projection (FBP) operation by learning a weighted combination of the different receptive sensors based on the signal collected from scattered light emitted at different locations in the reconstructed tissue. Empirically we did not observe any improvements in the reconstruction results using more than one fully connected layer. This may be related to the size of the input measurement which is only 256 dimensional in our dataset. Higher dimensional inputs may benefit from additional layers.

Convolutional Layers: A set of convolutional layers, with 64 channels, are used to refine the first image and produce the final reconstruction image. The non linear ReLU activation and zero-padding are employed at each convolution layer. All feature maps produced by all convolutional layers are set to size 128×128. The size of the convolution filters is increased gradually to cover a larger receptive field at deeper layers and capture local spacial correlations. Details of the architecture are shown in Fig. 2.

Integration Layer: The integration layer is a convolutional layer with 7×7 kernel size and a single output channel. It is used to reduce features across the channels from the penultimate layer of the CNN model into a single channel. The output of this layer is the reconstructed image.

Training: We trained the model by minimizing the mean squared error between the reconstructed image and the ground truth synthetic image. We used an L^2 norm penalty on the last convolutional layer output as it facilitates training (i.e. we observed faster convergence using regularization). The model was implemented in Keras and trained for a total of 2,000 epochs on an Nvidia Titan X GPU using batch gradient descent with momentum. The learning rate was set to 0.001 and we used a learning decay of 1e−6, momentum was set to 0.9. All training hyper-parameters were optimized via grid search on a validation set. We sequentially trained the model to first reconstruct an image using the fully connected layer only, then we fine-tuned the entire architecture after including the different convolution layers (Fig. 2).

Note that the model was only trained on synthetic data and we kept the phantom data for evaluation only, as depicted in Fig. 2. In total, we generated 4,500 synthetic training images and their corresponding simulated DOT measurements and tested our model in 200 synthetic DOT measurements then in 32 phantom real probe measurements with corresponding ground truth images.

3   Experiments and Results

We compared our results with those obtained by the analytic reconstruction approach described in [5]. Briefly, the analytic method is based on comparing the collected measurement to the measurement of a tissue-equivalent solution with homogeneous value. The resulting difference is then used to perform filtered back-projection and to estimate the spatial location of the lesion.

Qualitative Results: Once trained using the generated synthetic data, our model was tested on the phantom dataset. In Fig. 3, we visually compare our proposed reconstruction method to the analytic approach results for phantom cases. Evidently, the images reconstructed by our method are more accurate than those reconstructed by the more conventional analytic approach, when tested on data with a known ground truth. In Fig. 3 we show the reconstructed image using only the first fully connected layer which is equivalent to the filtered back-projection operation. Our qualitative results show that reconstructions obtained with one fully connected layer (third column in Fig. 3) are on par with reconstructions obtained with the analytic approach (second column in Fig. 3).

Quantitative Results: In order to measure the quality of the results, we consider the mean square error as well as the distance between the centre of the lesions in the ground truth image versus the reconstructed image. The peak signal to noise ratio (PSNR), the SSIM similarity measure, and the Jaccard index (intersection over union) are also calculated. The Jaccard index, used for comparing the similarity and diversity of sample sets, is the ratio of area of overlap between detected and ground truth lesion to the area of their union. This metric is computed after thresholding the reconstructed image to obtain a binary mask where foreground pixels correspond to pixels with highest optical coefficient.

Table 1 shows the results for the phantom dataset. This experiment also allows us to evaluate the quality of the synthetic dataset we generated by testing how well a model trained only on synthetic data generalizes to unseen physical phantom images. Results reported in Table 1 show that the proposed approach is able to generalize well to the phantom dataset and achieves better performance than the baseline analytic approach in terms of distance (+50%), Jaccard index

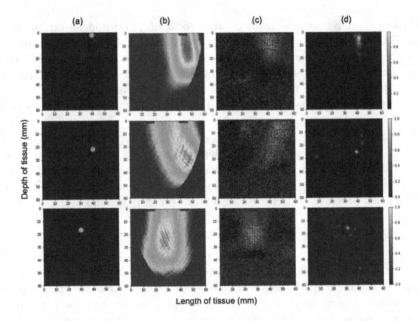

Fig. 3. Qualitative reconstruction performance of our model compared to conventional techniques. (a)–(d): Ground truth; analytic approach results; generalized FBP with one fully connected layer only; and proposed model results.

Table 1. Quantitative results scores on 32 phantom test measurements

	Distance (pixel)	MSE	PSNR (db)	SSIM	Jaccard	Time (ms)
Analytic approach	77.4 ± 32.2	0.06 ± 0.05	15.08 ± 6	0.32 ± 0.26	0.5 ± 0.19	83.3
Proposed model	33.2 ± 23.4	0.02 ± 0.03	20.1 ± 4.6	0.46 ± 0.28	0.85 ± 0.07	7.3

(+35%), similarity score (+14%) and PSNR (+5db). The high standard deviation in distance metric is mainly due to samples with deep lesion (lesion location ≥ 30 mm) since as the lesion depth increases it becomes harder to differentiate the signal from the tumor-free tissue signal. On average, our model achieves an order of magnitude faster reconstruction than the baseline analytic approach.

4   Conclusion

This work represents a step forward for both image reconstruction in DOT and the use of machine learning in bio-imaging. We present the first model that leverages physics based forward projection simulators to generate realistic synthetic datasets and we model the inverse problem with a deep learning model where the architecture is tailored to accurately reconstruct images from DOT measurement. We test the method on real acquired projection measurements subject to sensor non-idealities and noise. Results show that our method improves the quality of reconstructed images and shows promising results towards real-time image reconstruction. In future work, we will focus on exploring even more realistic DOT simulation scenarios and extend the study to clinical cases.

Acknowledgments. We thank NVIDIA Corporation for the donation of Titan X GPUs used in this research and the Natural Sciences and Engineering Research Council of Canada (NSERC) for partial funding.

References

1. Panieri, E.: Breast cancer screening in developing countries. Best Pract. Res. Clin. Obstet. Gynaecol. **26**, 283–290 (2012)
2. Godavarty, A., Rodriguez, S., Jung, Y.J., Gonzalez, S.: Optical imaging for breast cancer prescreening. Breast Cancer: Targets Ther. **7**, 193 (2015)
3. Shokoufi, M., Golnaraghi, F.: Development of a handheld diffuse optical breast cancer assessment probe. J. Innov. Opt. Health Sci. **9**(2), 1650007 (2016)
4. Flexman, M.L., Kim, H.K., Stoll, R., et al.: A wireless handheld probe with spectrally constrained evolution strategies for diffuse optical imaging of tissue. Rev. Sci. Instrum. **83**(3), 033108 (2012)
5. Shokoufi, M.: Multi-modality breast cancer assessment tools using diffuse optical and electrical impedance spectroscopy. Ph.D. thesis (2016)
6. Jin, K.H., McCann, M.T., Froustey, E., Unser, M.: Deep convolutional neural network for inverse problems in imaging. IEEE Trans. Image Process. **26**(9), 4509–4522 (2017)
7. Sidky, E.Y., Pan, X.: Image reconstruction in circular cone-beam computed tomography by constrained, total-variation minimization. Phys. Med. Biol. **53**(17), 4777 (2008)
8. Wang, G.: A perspective on deep imaging. IEEE Access **4**, 8914–8924 (2016)
9. Chen, H., et al.: Low-dose CT with a residual encoder-decoder convolutional neural network. IEEE Trans. Med. Imaging **36**(12), 2524–2535 (2017)
10. Schlemper, J., Caballero, J., Hajnal, J.V., Price, A., Rueckert, D.: A deep cascade of convolutional neural networks for MR image reconstruction. In: Niethammer, M. (ed.) IPMI 2017. LNCS, vol. 10265, pp. 647–658. Springer, Cham (2017). https://doi.org/10.1007/978-3-319-59050-9_51
11. McCann, M.T., Jin, K.H., Unser, M.: A review of convolutional neural networks for inverse problems in imaging. (2017). arXiv preprint arXiv:1710.04011
12. Boublil, D., Elad, M., Shtok, J., Zibulevsky, M.: Spatially-adaptive reconstruction in computed tomography using neural networks. IEEE Trans. Med. Imaging **34**(7), 1474–1485 (2015)
13. Nguyen, T.C., Bui, V., Nehmetallah, G.: Computational optical tomography using 3-D deep convolutional neural networks. Opt. Eng. **57**(4), 043111 (2018)
14. Zhu, B., Liu, J.Z., Cauley, S.F., Rosen, B.R., Rosen, M.S.: Image reconstruction by domain-transform manifold learning. Nature **555**(7697), 487 (2018)
15. Ghosh, N., Mohanty, S.K., Majumder, S.K., Gupta, P.K.: Measurement of optical transport properties of normal and malignant human breast tissue. Appl. Opt. **40**(1), 176–184 (2001)
16. Schweiger, M., Arridge, S.R.: The Toast++ software suite for forward and inverse modeling in optical tomography. J. Biomed. Opt. **19**(4), 040801 (2014)

Image Reconstruction via Variational Network for Real-Time Hand-Held Sound-Speed Imaging

Valery Vishnevskiy[✉], Sergio J. Sanabria, and Orcun Goksel

Computer-assisted Applications in Medicine Group, ETH Zurich, Zurich, Switzerland
vishnevskiy@biomed.ee.ethz.ch

Abstract. Speed-of-sound is a biomechanical property for quantitative tissue differentiation, with great potential as a new ultrasound-based image modality. A conventional ultrasound array transducer can be used together with an acoustic mirror, or so-called reflector, to reconstruct sound-speed images from time-of-flight measurements to the reflector collected between transducer element pairs, which constitutes a challenging problem of limited-angle computed tomography. For this problem, we herein present a variational network based image reconstruction architecture that is based on optimization loop unrolling, and provide an efficient training protocol of this network architecture on fully synthetic inclusion data. Our results indicate that the learned model presents good generalization ability, being able to reconstruct images with significantly different statistics compared to the training set. Complex inclusion geometries were shown to be successfully reconstructed, also improving over the prior-art by 23% in reconstruction error and by 10% in contrast on synthetic data. In a phantom study, we demonstrated the detection of multiple inclusions that were not distinguishable by prior-art reconstruction, meanwhile improving the contrast by 27% for a stiff inclusion and by 219% for a soft inclusion. Our reconstruction algorithm takes approximately 10 ms, enabling its use as a real-time imaging method on an ultrasound machine, for which we are demonstrating an example preliminary setup herein.

Keywords: Deep learning · Speed-of-sound · Image reconstruction

1 Introduction

Speed-of-sound (SoS) ultrasound computed tomography (USCT) is a promising image modality, which generates maps of speed of sound in tissue as an imaging biomarker. Potential clinical applications are differentiation of breast tumorous lesions [3], breast density assessment [13,15], staging of musculoskeletal [11] and non-alcoholic fatty liver disease [7], amongst others. For this, a set of time of flight (ToF) measurements through the tissue between pairs of transmit/receive elements of an ultrasonic array can be used for a tomographic reconstruction.

© Springer Nature Switzerland AG 2018
F. Knoll et al. (Eds.): MLMIR 2018, LNCS 11074, pp. 120–128, 2018.
https://doi.org/10.1007/978-3-030-00129-2_14

Various 2D ad 3D acquisition setups have been proposed, including circular or dome-shaped transducer geometries, which provide multilateral set of measurements that are convenient for reconstruction methods [8] but costly to manufacture and cumbersome in use. Hand-held reflector based setup [10,14] depicted in Fig. 1a uses a conventional portable ultrasound probe to measure ToF via wave reflections of a plate placed on the opposite side of the sample. Despite its simplicity, such a setup results in limited-angle (LA) CT, which requires prior assumptions and suitable regularization and numerical optimization techniques to produce meaningful reconstructions [14]. Such optimization techniques may not be guaranteed to converge, are often slow in runtime, and involve parameters that are difficult to set.

In this paper, we propose a problem-specific variational network [1,5] for limited-angle SoS reconstruction, with parameters learned from numerous forward simulations. Contrary to machine learning methods based on sinogram inpainting [16] and reconstruction artefact removal [6] for LA-CT, we learn reconstruction process end-to-end, and show that it allows to qualitatively improve conventional reconstruction.

2   Methods

Using the wave reflection tracking algorithm described in [14], we measure the ToF Δt between transmit (Tx) and receive (Rx) transducers in a $M = 128$ element linear ultrasound array (see Fig. 1a). Discretizing corresponding ray paths using a Gaussian sampling kernel, the inverse of ToF can be expressed as a linear combination of tissue slowness values x [s/m], i.e. $(\Delta t)^{-1} = \sum_{i \in \text{Ray}} l_i x_i$. Considering a Cartesian $n_1 \times n_2 = P$ grid, we define the forward model

$$\mathbf{b} = \text{diag}(\mathbf{m})\mathbf{L}\mathbf{x} + \mathcal{N}(\mathbf{0}, \sigma_N \mathbf{I}), \tag{1}$$

where $\mathbf{x} \in \mathbb{R}^P$ is the inverse SoS (slowness) map, $\mathbf{L} \in \mathbb{R}^{M^2 \times P}$ is a sparse path matrix defined by acquisition geometry and discretization scheme, $\mathbf{m} \in \{0, 1\}^{M^2}$ is the undersampling mask with zeros indicating a missing (e.g., unreliable) ToF measurement between a corresponding Tx-Rx pair, and $\mathbf{b} \in \mathbb{R}^{M^2}$ is a zero-filled vector of measured inverse ToFs $(\Delta t)^{-1}$. Reconstructing a slowness map $\mathbf{x}$ is a process inverse to (1) and can be posed as the following convex optimization problem:

$$\hat{\mathbf{x}}(\mathbf{b}, \mathbf{m}; \lambda, \boldsymbol{\nabla}) = \underset{\mathbf{x}}{\text{argmin}} \; \|\text{diag}(\mathbf{m})\mathbf{L}\mathbf{x} - \mathbf{b}\|_1 + \lambda \|\boldsymbol{\nabla}\mathbf{x}\|_1, \tag{2}$$

which we solve using ADMM [2] algorithm with Cholesky factorization. Here $\boldsymbol{\nabla}$ is a matrix, and λ is the regularization weight.

It is common to choose regularization matrix $\boldsymbol{\nabla}_{\text{TV}}$ that implements spatial gradients on Cartesian grid, yielding the total variation (TV) regularization [12], which allows to efficiently recover sharp image boundaries, but can introduce signal underestimation and staircase artefacts that are amplified by the limited-angle acquisition. In attempt to remedy this problem, one can delicately construct a set of image filters that will penalize problem-specific reconstruction artefacts. We follow [14] and use regularization matrix ∇_{MATV} that implements convolution with the set of weighted directional gradient operators. This weights regularization according to known wave path information, such that the locations with information from a narrower angular range are regularized more.

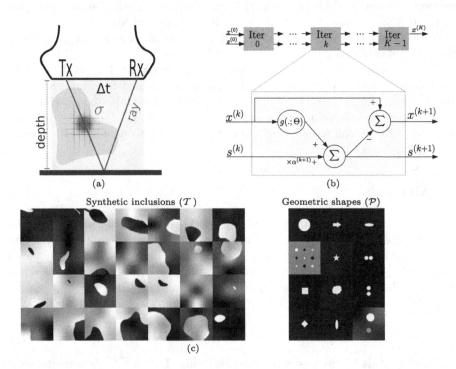

(a)

(b)

Synthetic inclusions ($\mathcal{T}$)

Geometric shapes ($\mathcal{P}$)

(c)

Fig. 1. (a) Acquisition setup and ray tracing discretization. (b) Structure of variational network; tunable parameters of the layer are highlighted in red. (c) Samples from synthetic training set $\mathcal{T}$ and testing set of geometric primitives $\mathcal{P}$. (Color figure online)

2.1   Variational Network

Variational networks (VN) is a class of deep learning methods that incorporate a parametrized prototype of a reconstruction algorithm in differentiable manner. A successful VN architecture proposed by Hammernik et al. in [5] for undersampled MRI reconstruction unrolls a fixed number of iterations of the gradient descent (GD) algorithm applied to a virtual optimization-based reconstruction problem. By unrolling the iterations of the algorithm into network layers (see Fig. 1b), the output is expressed as a formula parametrized by the regularization parameters and step lengths of this GD algorithm. The parameters are then tuned on retrospectively undersampled training data.

In contrast to discrete Fourier transform, the design matrix of LA-CT is poorly conditioned, which compromises the performance of conventional GD. Therefore, we propose to enhance the VN in the following ways: (i) unroll GD with momentum, (ii) add left diagonal preconditioner $\mathbf{p}^{(k)} \in \mathbb{R}^{M^2}$ for the path matrix $\mathbf{L}$, (iii) use adaptive data consistency term $\varphi_d^{(k)}$, and (iv) allow spatial filter weighting $\mathbf{w}_i^{(k)} \in \mathbb{R}^P$. The resulting reconstruction network is defined in Algorithm 1 with tunable parameters Θ, where each of K variational layers contains N_f convolution matrices $\mathbf{D} = \mathbf{D}(\mathbf{d})$ with $N_c \times N_c$ kernels $\mathbf{d}$ that are ensured to be zero-centered unit-norm via re-parametrization: $\mathbf{d} = (\mathbf{d}' - \langle \mathbf{d}' \rangle)/\|(\mathbf{d}' - \langle \mathbf{d}' \rangle)\|_2$, where $\langle . \rangle$ denotes mean value of the vector. Each filter $\mathbf{D}$ is associated with its potential function $\varphi_r\{.\}$ that is parametrized via cubic interpolation of control knots $\phi_r \in \mathbb{R}^{N_g}$ placed on Cartesian grid on $[-r, r]$ interval. Data term potentials $\varphi_d\{.\}$ are defined in the same way. The network is trained to minimize ℓ_1-norm of the reconstruction error on the training set $\mathcal{T}$:

$$\min_{\Theta} \ \mathbb{E}_{\{\mathbf{b},\mathbf{m},\mathbf{x}^\star\} \in \mathcal{T}} \|\mathcal{V}(\mathbf{b}, \mathbf{m}; \Theta) - \mathbf{x}^\star\|_1. \tag{3}$$

Input: $\mathbf{b}$ — inverse ToF, $\mathbf{m}$ — undersampling mask
Parameters: $\Theta = \{\phi_d^{(k)}, \phi_{r,i}^{(k)}, \mathbf{p}^{(k)}, \mathbf{w}_i^{(k)}, \mathbf{D}_i^{(k)}, \alpha^{(k)}\}_{i=1,\dots,N_f,\ k=1,\dots,K}$
$\mathbf{x}^{(0)} \leftarrow \alpha^{(0)} \mathbf{L}^\mathsf{T} \mathbf{b}, \quad \mathbf{s}^{(0)} \leftarrow \mathbf{0}$
for $k := 0$ to $K - 1$
  $\mathbf{g}^{(k)} \leftarrow \mathbf{L}^\mathsf{T} \mathrm{diag}(\mathbf{p}^{(k)})\mathrm{diag}(\mathbf{m})\, \varphi_d^{(k)} \left\{ \mathrm{diag}(\mathbf{m})\mathrm{diag}(\mathbf{p}^{(k)}) \left(\mathbf{L}\mathbf{x}^{(k)} - \mathbf{b} \right) \right\} +$
    $\sum_{i=1,\dots,N_f} \left(\mathbf{D}_i^{(k)}\right)^\mathsf{T} \mathrm{diag}(\mathbf{w}_i^{(k)})\, \varphi_{r,i}^{(k)} \left\{ \mathrm{diag}(\mathbf{w}_i^{(k)})\mathbf{D}_i^{(k)}\mathbf{x}^{(k)} \right\}$
  $\mathbf{s}^{(k+1)} \leftarrow \alpha^{(k+1)}\mathbf{s}^{(k)} + \mathbf{g}^{(k)}$
  $\mathbf{x}^{(k+1)} \leftarrow \mathbf{x}^{(k)} - \mathbf{s}^{(k+1)}$
Output: reconstructed image $\mathcal{V}(\mathbf{b}, \mathbf{m}; \Theta) := \mathbf{x}^{(K)}$

Algorithm 1: Proposed variational reconstruction network model VNv4.

Training. Dataset $\mathcal{T}$ is generated using fixed acquisition geometry with reflector depth equal to transducer array width. High-resolution (HR) 256×256 synthetic inclusion masks are produced by applying smooth deformation to an ellipse with random center, eccentricity, and radius. Two smooth slowness maps with random values from $[1/1650, 1/1350]$ interval are then blended with this inclusion mask, yielding a final slowness map $\mathbf{x}_{HR}^\star$ (see Fig. 1c). The chosen range corresponds to observed SoS values for breast tissues of different densities and tumorous inclusions of different pathologies [4]. Forward path matrix $\mathbf{L}_{HR}$ and random incoherent undersmapling mask $\mathbf{m}$ are used to generate noisy inverse ToF vector $\mathbf{b}$ according to model (1) with $\sigma_N = 2 \cdot 10^{-8}$. Finally, we downsample $\mathbf{x}_{HR}^\star$ to $n_1 \times n_2$ size yielding the ground truth map $\mathbf{x}^\star$. About 10% of maps did not contain inclusions. For each reconstruction problem the path matrix $\mathbf{L}$ is normalized with its largest singular value, and inverse ToF are centered and scaled: $\mathbf{b}' = \mathbf{b} - (\langle \mathbf{b} \rangle / \langle \mathbf{L1} \rangle)\mathbf{L1}, \ \tilde{\mathbf{b}} = \mathbf{b}'/\mathrm{std}(\mathbf{b}')$.

The configuration of networks were the following: $K = 10$, $N_f = 50$, $N_c = 5$, $n_1 = n_2 = 64$, $N_g = 55$. All parameters were initialized from $\mathcal{U}(0, 1)$. We refer to this architecture as VNv4. Ablating spatial filter weighting $\mathbf{w}_i^{(k)}$ from VNv4, we get VNv3; additionally ablating adaptive data potentials $\varphi_d^{(k)}$, we get VNv2; further ablating preconditioner $\mathbf{p}^{(k)}$, we get VNv1; and eventually unrolling GD without momentum, VNv0. For tuning the aforementioned models we used 10^5 iterations of Adam algorithm [9] with learning rate 10^{-3} and batch size 25. Every 5000 iterations we readjust potential function's interval range r by setting it to the maximal observed value of the corresponding activation function argument.

3   Results

We compare TV and MA-TV against VN architectures on (i) 200 samples from $\mathcal{T}$ that were set aside and unseen during training, and (ii) a set $\mathcal{P}$ of 14 geometric primitives depicted in Fig. 1c, using following metrics:

$$\text{SAD}(\mathbf{x}, \mathbf{y}) = \frac{\|\mathbf{x} - \mathbf{y}\|_1}{P}, \quad \text{CR} = \frac{2\left|\mu_{\text{inc}} - \mu_{\text{bg}}\right|}{\left|\mu_{\text{inc}}\right| + \left|\mu_{\text{bg}}\right|}, \quad \text{CRf} = \frac{\text{estimated CR}}{\text{ground truth CR}}, \quad (4)$$

where μ_{inc} and μ_{bg} are mean values in the inclusion and background regions accordingly. The optimal regularization weight λ for TV and MA-TV algorithms was tuned to give the best (lowest) SAD on the P3 image (see Fig. 2). Similarly to training generation, the forward model for validation and test sets was computed on high resolution images with normal noise and 30% undersmapling.

Quantitative evaluation on synthetic data is reported in Table 1 and shows that the proposed VNv4 network outperforms conventional TV and MA-TV reconstruction methods both in terms of accuracy and contrast. Comparing VNv options, it can be seen that richer architectures performed better. Figure 2 shows qualitative evaluation of reconstruction methods. VNv4 is able to reconstruct multiple inclusions (P5), handle smooth SoS variation (T1), and generally maintain inclusion position and geometry without hallucinating nonexistent inclusions. Although for some geometries (e.g. P4) TV reconstruction has lower SAD value, VNv4 provides better contrast, which allows to separate the two inclusions. As expected from the limited-angle nature of the data, highly elongated inclusions that are parallel to the reflector either undergo axial geometric distortion (P1), or could not be adequately reconstructed (T3) by any presented method.

Breast Phantom Experiment. We also compared the reconstruction methods using a realistic breast elastography phantom (Model 059, CIRS Inc.) that mimics glandular tissue with two lesions of different density. Portable ultrasound system (UF-760AG, Fukuda Denshi Inc., Tokyo, Japan) streams full-matrix RF ultrasound data over a high bandwidth link to a dedicated PC, which is used to perform USCT reconstruction and output a live SoS video feedback (cf. Fig. 4).

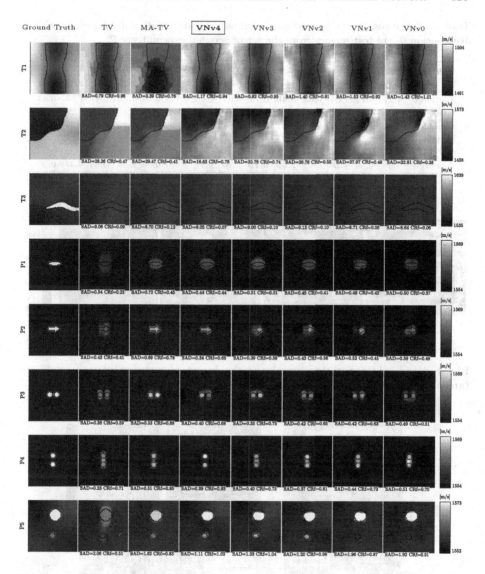

Fig. 2. Sound speed reconstructions of synthetic data from sets $\mathcal{T}$, $\mathcal{P}$ and single natural image N1. Inclusions are delineated with red curves. For each image transducer array is placed on top and reflector on bottom. (Color figure online)

We used an ultrasound probe (FUT-LA385-12P) with 128 piezoelectric transducer elements. For each frame a total of 128×128 RF lines are generated for all Tx/Rx combinations, at an imaging center frequency of 5 MHz digitized at 40.96 MHz. As seen in Fig. 3, VNv4 qualitatively outperforms both TV and MA-TV methods, showing clearly distinguishable hard and soft lesions. Run-time of MA-TV and TV algorithms on CPU is $\sim$30 s per image, while VN reconstruction takes $\sim$0.4 s on CPU and $\sim$0.01 s on GPU.

Table 1. SoS reconstruction measures computed on 200 validation images from training distribution $\mathcal{T}$, 14 test images from the set of geometric primitives $\mathcal{P}$.

Shape set	TV		MA-TV		VNv4		VNv3		VNv2		VNv1		VNv0	
	SAD	CRf	SAD	CRf	SAD	CRf	SAD	CRf	SAD	CRf	SAD	CRf	SAD	CRf
Synthetic inc. ($\mathcal{T}$)	7.27	0.49	7.64	0.53	**5.46**	**0.71**	5.91	0.66	6.77	0.59	7.56	0.47	7.96	0.43
Geometric shapes ($\mathcal{P}$)	0.54	0.63	0.72	0.84	**0.51**	**0.79**	0.60	0.77	0.62	0.73	0.77	0.60	0.78	0.57
Average	3.90	0.56	4.18	0.68	**2.99**	**0.75**	3.26	0.71	3.69	0.66	4.16	0.53	4.37	0.50

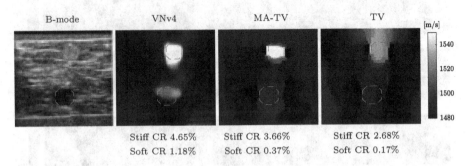

B-mode   VNv4   MA-TV   TV   [m/s]

1540

1520

1500

1480

Stiff CR 4.65%   Stiff CR 3.66%   Stiff CR 2.68%
Soft CR 1.18%   Soft CR 0.37%   Soft CR 0.17%

Fig. 3. Hand-held SoS mammography of the breast phantom. Stiff (red) and soft (green) inclusions were delineated in the B-mode image. (Color figure online)

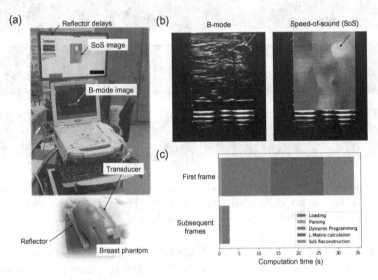

Fig. 4. Live SoS imaging demonstration. (a) Experimental setup. (b) Sample outputs of B-mode and SoS video feedback. A non-echogenic stiff lesion is clearly delineated in the SoS image. (c) Computational benchmarks, also showing initialization and memory allocation times. After initialization, SoS reconstruction time is negligible compared to data transfer and reflector ToF measurement via dynamic programming [14].

4   Discussion

In this paper we have proposed a deep variational reconstruction network for hand-held US sound-speed imaging. The method is able to reconstruct various inclusion geometries both in synthetic and phantom experiments. VN demonstrated good generalization ability, which suggests that unrolling even more sophisticated numerical schemes may be possible. Improvements over conventional reconstruction algorithms are both qualitative and quantitative. The ability of method to distinguish hard and soft inclusions has great diagnostic potential in characterizing lesions in real-time.

References

1. Adler, J., Öktem, O.: Solving ill-posed inverse problems using iterative deep neural networks. Inverse Probl. **33**(12), 124007 (2017)
2. Boyd, S., Parikh, N., Chu, E., Peleato, B., Eckstein, J.: Distributed optimization and statistical learning via the alternating direction method of multipliers. Found. Trends ML **3**(1), 1–122 (2011)
3. Duric, N., et al.: In-vivo imaging results with ultrasound tomography: report on an on-going study at the Karmanos cancer institute. In: SPIE Med Imaging, pp. 76290M–1/M–9 (2010)
4. Duric, N., et al.: Detection of breast cancer with ultrasound tomography: first results with the computed ultrasound risk evaluation (cure) prototype. Med. Phys. **34**(2), 773–785 (2007)
5. Hammernik, K., Klatzer, T., Kobler, E., Recht, M.P., Sodickson, D.K., Pock, T., Knoll, F.: Learning a variational network for reconstruction of accelerated MRI data. MRM **79**, 3055–3071 (2018)
6. Hammernik, K., Würfl, T., Pock, T., Maier, A.: A deep learning architecture for limited-angle computed tomography reconstruction. Bildverarbeitung für die Medizin **2017**, 92–97 (2017)
7. Imbault, M., et al.: Robust sound speed estimation for ultrasound-based hepatic steatosis assessment. Phys. Med. Biol. **62**(9), 3582 (2017)
8. Jirik, R., et al.: Sound-speed image reconstruction in sparse-aperture 3-D ultrasound transmission tomography. IEEE Trans. Ultrason. Ferroelectr. Freq. Control **59**(2) (2012)
9. Kingma, D.P., Ba, J.: Adam: a method for stochastic optimization. arXiv preprint arXiv:1412.6980 (2014)
10. Krueger, M., Burow, V., Hiltawsky, K., Ermert, H.: Limited angle ultrasonic transmission tomography of the compressed female breast. In: Ultrasonics Symposium, vol. 2, pp. 1345–1348. IEEE (1998)
11. Qu, X., et al.: Limb muscle sound speed estimation by ultrasound computed tomography excluding receivers in bone shadow. In: SPIE Medical Imaging, p. 101391 (2017)
12. Rudin, L., Osher, S., Fatemi, E.: Nonlinear total variation based noise removal algorithms. Physica D: Nonlinear Phenomena **60**(1–4), 259–268 (1992)
13. Sak, M., et al.: Comparison of breast density measurements made with ultrasound tomography and mammography. In: SPIE Medical Imaging, pp. 94190R–1/R–8 (2015)

14. Sanabria, S.J., Goksel, O.: Hand-held sound-speed imaging based on ultrasound reflector delineation. In: Ourselin, S., Joskowicz, L., Sabuncu, M.R., Unal, G., Wells, W. (eds.) MICCAI 2016. LNCS, vol. 9900, pp. 568–576. Springer, Cham (2016). https://doi.org/10.1007/978-3-319-46720-7_66
15. Sanabria, S.J., et al.: Breast-density assessment with hand-held ultrasound: a novel biomarker to assess breast cancer risk and to tailor screening? Eur. Radiol. (2018)
16. Tovey, R., et al.: Directional sinogram inpainting for limited angle tomography. arXiv preprint arXiv:1804.09991 (2018)

Towards Arbitrary Noise Augmentation—Deep Learning for Sampling from Arbitrary Probability Distributions

Felix Horger, Tobias Würfl, Vincent Christlein, and Andreas Maier[✉]

Pattern Recognition Lab of the Friedrich-Alexander-University Erlangen-Nuremberg,
Erlangen, Germany
andreas.maier@fau.de

Abstract. Accurate noise modelling is important for training of deep learning reconstruction algorithms. While noise models are well known for traditional imaging techniques, the noise distribution of a novel sensor may be difficult to determine a priori. Therefore, we propose learning arbitrary noise distributions. To do so, this paper proposes a fully connected neural network model to map samples from a uniform distribution to samples of any explicitly known probability density function. During the training, the Jensen-Shannon divergence between the distribution of the model's output and the target distribution is minimized.

We experimentally demonstrate that our model converges towards the desired state. It provides an alternative to existing sampling methods such as inversion sampling, rejection sampling, Gaussian mixture models and Markov-Chain-Monte-Carlo. Our model has high sampling efficiency and is easily applied to any probability distribution, without the need of further analytical or numerical calculations.

1 Introduction

Accurate physical modelling is very important for deep learning reconstruction methods [1]. Therefore, accurate augmentation is a must. Typically, this is performed by sampling from a given probability density function (PDF). Existing methods for generating such samples include inversion sampling, rejection sampling, Gaussian mixture or Markov-Chain-Monte-Carlo methods. In any case, random samples of a distribution easy to sample from, such as a uniform distribution, are used to generate samples of the desired distribution. However, in very new imaging techniques analytical derivation of accurate noise models is difficult and thus the noise model may be unknown. As a result, applying deep learning methods trained on simulation data to real scanners is a challenge [2].

In this paper, we examine how a fully connected neural network (FCNN) model performs on generating random numbers of a given distribution. Our model is constructed to map an input vector consisting of n samples from a uniform distribution to an output vector with the same dimension. For training,

© Springer Nature Switzerland AG 2018
F. Knoll et al. (Eds.): MLMIR 2018, LNCS 11074, pp. 129–137, 2018.
https://doi.org/10.1007/978-3-030-00129-2_15

we merely need a noise source that is able to generate random numbers of the given distribution. Such a model yields the highest possible sampling efficiency since n input samples are required to generate n output samples. It is flexible towards the choice of the target PDF and needs little manual effort.

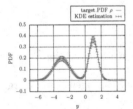 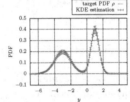 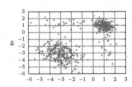

(a) Average of 500 KDEs each from 500 random values produced with the mixture of Gaussians method.

(b) Mean of the KDE of 500 output vectors, each consisting of 500 elements. The training was performed on $5 \cdot 10^6$ input vectors.

(c) Two randomly chosen elements of 500 output vectors plotted against each other, showing the dependence of the model's output values.

Fig. 1. Comparison of the model to the mixture of Gaussians method on a bimodal Gaussian target, given by Eq. (4).

2 Conventional Sampling Methods

2.1 Inversion Sampling

This method provides a function, which maps samples from an arbitrary distribution $\alpha(x)$ to samples from the target PDF $\rho(y)$. Let $\varphi\colon x \mapsto y$ be this function, then, assuming that φ is a bijection, the differential equation

$$\alpha(x)\,\mathrm{d}x = \rho(\varphi(x))\,\mathrm{d}\varphi \tag{1}$$

holds. If α is the uniform distribution over $[0,1]$, then φ can be determined to be equal to the inverse cumulative distribution function (CDF) corresponding to ρ. In many cases, the CDF or its inverse might not have an analytical representation. If the integration and inversion are performed numerically, the computational effort increases and the quality of the samples decreases. In contrast, if φ is explicitly known, this method has high efficiency and produces samples with exactly the desired properties. If the samples drawn from α are independent, the same holds for the produced samples.

This method may be applied to higher dimensional PDFs, using either the separability of PDFs of uncorrelated random variables or the Bayes' theorem for correlated random variables, to split the sampling process into multiple one-dimensional sampling steps. For this approach all the conditional one-dimensional PDFs have to be known [3, 526ff].

2.2   Rejection Sampling

This method requires a proposal distribution $\beta(y)$ from which sampling can be performed. Additionally, a constant c such that $c \cdot \beta(y) \geq \rho(y) \; \forall y$ is required.

The procedure starts with drawing a sample y from β and another sample r from the uniform distribution R over $[0, c \cdot \beta(y)]$. If $r < \rho(y)$, then y is a valid sample from ρ, otherwise y is rejected. This process is continued until enough valid samples have been generated.

The major disadvantage of this method is that sampling efficiency depends on how close the proposal distribution lies to the target distribution. Besides that, the produced samples are independent samples from ρ, if the samples drawn from β and R are independent. An advantage is that the target does not have to be normalized [3, 528ff].

2.3   Mixture of Gaussians

The quality of the samples produces by this method depends on how well a suitable sum of Gaussians approximates the target. Samples from the approximation can be obtained by randomly choosing a Gaussian mode from the sum with probability proportional to its weight and generating a sample from it.

This method is easy to perform since sampling from a Gaussian PDF can be done using inversion sampling and if the Gaussian samples are independent, the generated samples are independent as well [3, 110ff].

2.4   Markov-Chain-Monte-Carlo

The aim of this method is to construct a Markov chain with a stationary distribution equal to the target. The Metropolis-Hastings algorithm is a commonly used method of doing so. An initial sample y_0 is used to propose a possible next sample y', drawn from an arbitrary conditional distribution $q(y'|y_0)$. The sample is accepted as y_1, if

$$r \leq \min \left\{ 1, \; \frac{\rho(y')}{\rho(y_0)} \cdot \frac{q(y_0|y')}{q(y'|y_0)} \right\} \tag{2}$$

where r is drawn from the uniform distribution over $[0, 1]$. If y' is rejected, y_1 is equal to $y_{1-1} = y_0$. This is continued, until enough samples were obtained.

The proposal distribution $q(y'|y)$ has a great impact on the convergence of the distribution of the samples towards the target distribution. Consider for example a target with two modes placed distant to each other and a narrow proposal distribution located at y. It is very unlikely to switch between the modes, leading to slow convergence. Further, the initial sample y_0 has impact on the convergence: if $\rho(y_0)$ is small, it might need some time to reach areas of higher probability ("burn in"). As, the next sample is generated using the last one, the samples depend on each other [3, 539ff].

There is a possibility to link Markov-chain-Monte-Carlo methods and generative adversarial networks [4] in order to produce random numbers [5].

The generator is used as the transition kernel of the Markov chain if samples from the target distribution are accessible during the training. If this is not the case, the generator is trained to propose samples y'. Again, the proposal distribution has a great impact on the convergence and also the correlation of samples, thus this method is optimizing the step of proposing, leading to fast convergence and low correlation.

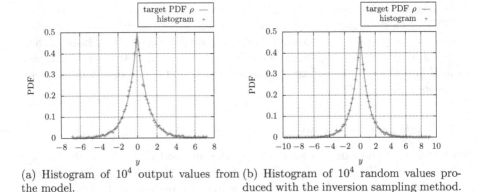

(a) Histogram of 10^4 output values from the model.

(b) Histogram of 10^4 random values produced with the inversion sampling method.

Fig. 2. Comparison of the model to the inversion sampling method on an exponential target given by Eq. (5).

2.5 FCNN Sampling

Our model is a simple FCNN, which is able to map an input vector consisting of n samples from the input distribution to an output vector of the same dimension. The target has to be known. The term "sample" refers in this context only to an element of any in- or output vector and is not to be understood as a "sample from the training set".

The model has n units in any layer and exponential linear unit (ELU) activation [6] in each but the last layer. A number of layers equal to ten has proven to lead to good results. The input dimension is $n = 500$, limited by the resources of the used hardware.

The ADAM optimizer [7] was used for the training process, the weights were initialized using the Xavier Glorot uniform distribution [8] and the biases were set to zero. The models were implemented using Python and Keras [9] with TensorFlow [10] backend. The loss-function of the model consists of three parts. The kernel density estimation (KDE) [11] of each output vector in a mini-batch is compared to the target. Additionally, the i-th element from each output vector in a mini-batch is extracted, treated as a set samples and its KDE is compared to the target. This performed for all i. It promotes diversity, otherwise the model produces the same output vector with the correct distribution for any input.

The comparison of the KDE and the target may be done using the mean-squared-error or the Jensen-Shannon-divergence [12], it was empirically found

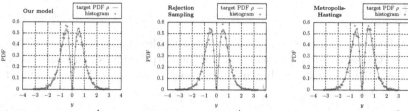

(a) Histogram of 10^4 output values from our model.

(b) Histogram of 10^4 random values produced with the rejection sampling method.

(c) Histogram of 10^4 random values produced with the Metropolis-Hastings algorithm.

Fig. 3. Comparison of our model to rejection sampling and the Metropolis-Hastings algorithm on the target given by Eq. (6).

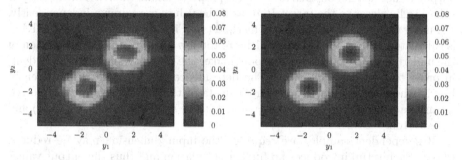

(a) 2D KDE of 10^4 output values from the model.

(b) The two-dimensional bimodal Gaussian target PDF.

Fig. 4. Comparison of the final KDE of our model's output values to the two-dimensional bimodal Gaussian target.

that the latter yields better results for most cases. The Jensen-Shannon-divergence

$$D_{JS}(p, q) = \frac{1}{2} \int_{\mathbb{R}} \left[p(y) \log \frac{p(y)}{q(y)} + q(y) \log \frac{q(y)}{p(y)} \right] dy \qquad (3)$$

between the PDFs p and q measures their similarity. The above integral has to approximated numerically, which is possible due to the properties of p and q. It is calculated on a finite set of discrete values. The third part of the loss-function to confines the output values in between the borders of this set using a "potential well", which was chosen to have linearly increasing sides.

The uniform distribution over $[-1, 1]$ was used to generate input samples. Any input distribution with zero mean leads to equal results, other distributions perform significantly worse. This is caused by the internal covariate shift, since no batch normalization was used for our model [13].

3   Results

Using this setup, our model is able to produce samples of a known target distribution, i. e., the kernel density estimation of the output values converges towards the target PDF. The input dimension is equal to 500 and the model has ten layers. The target is

$$\rho(y) = \frac{2 \cdot \exp\left[2 \cdot (x-1)^2\right] + \exp\left[\frac{1}{2}(x+3)^2\right]}{2\sqrt{2\pi}} \tag{4}$$

which is a bimodal asymmetric Gaussian. The resulting KDE of the output values is shown in Fig. 1b.

Since 500 values are fed at once into the network, it may happen that the output values depend on each other. This property allows the KDE of the output values to lie closer to the target PDF as if the values were drawn independently, e.g. using the mixture of Gaussians method (see Fig. 1a). Consider that the KDE is calculated of only 500 values, which are too few for a reasonable estimation of the underlying PDF. In fact, the model makes the output values interdependent, in order to overcome this issue. The dependence can be more clearly seen in Fig. 1, where two randomly chosen elements of the output vectors are plotted against each other. If they are independent, there would be peaks at $(-3, 1)$ and $(1, -3)$, too.

If independent samples are required, the input dimension may be reduced to one. Such setup introduces no further correlation and thus the output values are independent if the input values are independent as well. The model used in this scenario has 500 units per layer and ten layers. We can shown experimentally that the model with input dimension one represents the mapping function given by the inversion sampling method. This is not surprising because the differential equation Eq. (1) has a single solution on every finite subset of $\mathbb{R}$, given any boundary condition (Picard-Lindelöf theorem, note that there exist other mapping functions, which are not bijections, see Sect. 2.1).

The model with input dimension one was compared to the inversion sampling method for the target

$$\rho(y) = \frac{1}{2} \exp(-|y|) \tag{5}$$

an exponential distribution with extended domain $D = \mathbb{R}$. The training was performed on 10^7 input values and the histogram displayed in Fig. 2a was calculated out of 10^4 output values. In contrast, Fig. 2b shows the histogram of just as many random values obtained from the inversion sampling method.

Comparing these two yields no difference except that in Fig. 2b higher values occur. This may have been caused by the numerical precision and a more complicated fitting at the borders, since the model is represented by a continuous function, but the inverse CDF diverges at zero and one. This model was further compared to the rejection sampling method with a target

$$\rho(y) \propto y^2 \cdot \exp(-b|y|) \quad \text{with} \quad b > 0 \tag{6}$$

that has an inverse CDF with no analytical representation. Figure 3a shows the resulting histogram of 10^4 output values after a training on 10^7 input values. Comparatively, the histogram of the same amount of values produced with the rejection sampling method is displayed in Fig. 3b. The proposal distribution was chosen to be equal to Eq. (5). This is not the best choice since it has its maximum where the target is zero. Note that a bimodal Gaussian proposal can not be used since no constant c fulfills the condition given in Sect. 2.2. But a poor choice of the proposal distribution does not affect the quality of the samples, only the computational effort.

Comparing Fig. 3a and b yields that the histogram of the samples produced by our model approximates the target as well as samples produced with the rejection sampling method.

The same target was used for the Metropolis-Hastings algorithm, the proposal distribution was chosen to be a Gaussian with standard deviation 0.5 located at the current sample. As in Fig. 3c depicted, the histogram of the samples approximates the target and the goodness of the fit is comparable to Figs. 3a and b.

Further, the model is able to sample from two-dimensional PDFs of dependent variables. The model was trained on $2 \cdot 10^8$ input samples for a 2D bimodal Gaussian target with peaks at $(\pm 1.5, \pm 1.5)$ and variances of one in each direction. The result together with the target is depicted in Fig. 4.

The computational effort for the comparison of the estimation of output distribution and the target scales exponentially with the dimension. So there is a trade-off between training time and correct PDF-estimation. A possible solution is to manually split the PDF into its conditional one-dimensional parts and train a separate model for each dimension.

4   Conclusion

Summarizing this paper, our FCNN model is able to sample from any target PDF. The presented findings show that our model produces results with a goodness of the fit comparable to any existing sampling method. The quality of the approximation can be tuned using the model size and the training duration.

In order to apply our model, a noise source is required, in contrast to the Metropolis-Hastings algorithm or the rejection sampling method. On the other side, no proposal distribution, constant c (rejection sampling) or location of Gaussian modes (Gaussian mixture) has to be determined for our model. The only parameter of our model that has to be adjusted by hand is the width of the kernel function for the KDE of the output values.

Our model has the highest possible sampling efficiency equal to the inversion sampling method. Whereas the other described methods transform multiple samples into a single one. Especially the rejection sampling method may have low sampling efficiency.

Another important advantage is the flexibility towards the choice of the target. Compared to inversion sampling, no integration or inversion is required, neither analytical nor numerical. Our model with input dimension one tries to represent the inverse CDF. This is possible, as FCNN models are universal function approximators. It is neither required to choose how to proceed with the inversion, nor being bound to an approximation with Gaussian modes.

For high input dimensions, our model is able to generate dependent samples such that their distribution converges faster towards the target than the distribution of independent samples would do. If the input dimension is set to one, our model is able to produce independent samples if the input values are independent as well. This makes it more attractive than the Metropolis-Hastings algorithm, which produces highly dependent values and may have slow convergence.

Sampling from two-dimensional PDFs of dependent variables is also possible, but the curse of dimensionality has not yet been overcome. Splitting the target into conditional one-dimensional distributions using Bayes' theorem is a possible solution. Thus, we believe that neural networks are generally suited to learn noise distributions for data augmentation in deep learning image reconstruction.

References

1. Huang, Y., Würfl, T., Breininger, K., Liu, L., Lauritsch, G., Maier, A.: Some investigations on robustness of deep learning in limited angle tomography. In: Medical Image Computing and Computer-assisted Intervention (MICCAI) 2018, Granada, Spain, 16–20 September 2018 (2018, to appear)
2. Hoppe, E., et al.: Deep learning for magnetic resonance fingerprinting: a new approach for predicting quantitative parameter values from time series. In: German Medical Data Sciences: Visions and Bridges (62. Jahrestagung der GMDS) 2017, Oldenburg, Germany, 17–21 September 2017, pp. 202–206 (2017)
3. Bishop, C.M.: Pattern Recognition and Machine Learning (Information Science and Statistics). Springer, New York (2006)
4. Goodfellow, I.J., et al.: Generative adversarial networks (2014). http://arxiv.org/abs/1406.2661
5. Song, J., Zhao, S., Ermon, S.: A-NICE-MC: adversarial training for MCMC (2017). http://arxiv.org/abs/1706.07561
6. Clevert, D.A., Unterthiner, T., Hochreiter, S.: Fast and accurate deep network learning by exponential linear units (ELUs) (2015). http://arxiv.org/abs/1511.07289
7. Kingma, D.P., Ba, J.: Adam: a method for stochastic optimization (2014). http://arxiv.org/abs/1412.6980
8. Glorot, X., Bengio, Y.: Understanding the difficulty of training deep feedforward neural networks. In: Proceedings of the Thirteenth International Conference on Artificial Intelligence and Statistics, AISTATS 2010, Chia Laguna Resort, Sardinia, Italy, 13–15 May 2010, pp. 249–256 (2015)
9. Chollet, F., et al.: Keras (2015). https://github.com/fchollet/keras
10. Abadi, M., Agarwal, A., Barham, P., et al.: TensorFlow: large-scale machine learning on heterogeneous systems (2015). https://www.tensorflow.org/
11. Silverman, B.: Density Estimation for Statistics and Data Analysis. Chapman & Hall/CRC, London (1986)

12. Endres, D.M., Schindelin, J.E.: A new metric for probability distributions. IEEE Trans. Inf. Theory. **49**(7), 1858–1860 (2003)
13. Ioffe, S., Szegedy, C.: Batch normalization: accelerating deep network training by reducing internal covariate shift (2015). http://arxiv.org/abs/1502.03167

Left Atria Reconstruction from a Series of Sparse Catheter Paths Using Neural Networks

Alon Baram[1,2(✉)], Moshe Safran[3], Avi Ben-Cohen[1], and Hayit Greenspan[1]

[1] Faculty of Engineering, Department of Biomedical Engineering,
Medical Image Processing Laboratory, Tel Aviv University, 69978 Tel Aviv, Israel
alontbst@gmail.com
[2] Biosense Webster (Israel), Ltd. 4 Hatnufa Street, 20692 Yokneam, Israel
[3] RSIP Vision, 16 King George, 94229 Jerusalem, Israel

Abstract. Modeling and reconstructing the shape of a heart chamber from partial or noisy data is useful in many (minimally) invasive heart procedures. We propose a method to reconstruct the shape of the left atria during the electrophysiology procedure from a series of simple catheter maneuvers. We use left atria shapes generated from a statistical based physical model and approximate traversal locations of catheter maneuvers inside the left atria. These paths mimic realistic ones doable in a lab phantom. We demonstrate the ability of a deep neural network to approximate the atria shape solely based on the given paths. We compare the results against training from partial data generated by the intersection of a randomly generated sphere and the atria. We test the presented network on actual lab phantoms and show promising results.

Keywords: Minimally invasive electrophysiology
Left atria reconstruction · Deep neural network

1 Introduction and Related Work

Cardiac arrhythmia is a group of clinical conditions in which the heartbeat is irregular. Catheter ablation guided by electro-anatomic mapping (using CARTO or similar 3D mapping system) is one of the major invasive treatment choices for cardiac arrhythmia. Current systems map the geometry and electric signals by sampling points during catheter traversal of the chamber. After a significant amount of sampled points, a geometric reconstruction algorithm creates a surface that represents the boundary between blood pool and heart tissue. This surface is used to compute the electrical-chemical propagation wave that creates the chamber contraction. Figure 1a shows this map and irregular activity that can help to create an ablation strategy. Figure 1b shows the left atria (LA) anatomy and a common ablation procedure. Note the pulmonary veins (PV) names and structure (LI - left inferior, LS - left superior, RI - right inferior and RS - right superior).

© Springer Nature Switzerland AG 2018
F. Knoll et al. (Eds.): MLMIR 2018, LNCS 11074, pp. 138–146, 2018.
https://doi.org/10.1007/978-3-030-00129-2_16

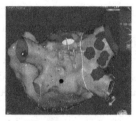 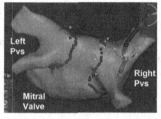

(a) LA electric propaga-
tion map

(b) LA physiology and typical
ablation (red points)

Fig. 1. Clinical use of LA surface (Color figure online)

The surface can be extracted using data gathered from other imaging devices such as MRI, Intra-cardiac ultrasonic catheters etc. A segmentation step is required to infer the boundary surface from the data acquired by the imaging modality. All systems suffer from at least some of the following limitations: noise, limited field of view (e.g. partially visited areas) and the change of the heart shape in real time and as a function of patient pose. To solve the segmentation problem, the gathered data from any imaging modality represents some function of how probable a point is to be a blood pool or in a tissue. The physician expects to see a smooth extracted shape with known anatomical parts and common proportions and orientations as the output of this segmentation.

In this work we develop a statistical model based approach using a neural network, to capture these requirements. Since patient atrium data (from CT or MRI) is not available, we use an existing model, developed by Biosense Webster [1] which is capable of generating likely left atria shapes. This is backed by a statistical model that is able to determine if the generated atria is probable. By using such a model we can generate examples of atria and teach a neural network to represent it. Using the learned representation it is our hope that meaningful de-noising and reconstruction from partial/noisy data can be learned.

Recent works use networks for complex shape modeling: In [2] a deep network is shown capable of representing 3D shapes and reconstructing them from partial data; [3] Used an auto-encoder to train a 2D CNN to detect and segment the left ventricle in an MRI image. There are several NNs in the literature that can generate instances from data, such as auto-encoders [4]. In [5], the authors generate 3D volumes of different shapes and interpolate between them using a variational auto-encoder [6] combined with a convolutional neural network (CNN).

In the current work we use a de-noising auto-encoder network to complete a left atria model from partial data, where some regions (large portions) of the data are missing. Our goal is to provide an accurate atria model in existing regions and a probable guess in missing regions. This simulates a stage in a real procedure where the physician visited a certain region of the atria and wants a visual estimate of the full atria. In Sect. 3.1 we generate a random sphere and intersect it with the atria. We learn the desired network architecture by reconstructing this partial data. In Sect. 3.2 we simulate a series of maneuvers that could be taken by the physician, train the model and reconstruct the Left Atria based on them. We feed synthetic path as input to model trained based on sphere intersection and compare results. Section 3.3 shows reconstruction results from data recorded in a lab phantom using an electromagnetic tracking system.

2   Methods

We train a de-noising auto-encoder with one or several hidden layers for our data completion tasks. The input and output are binary 3D volumes of size 30^3 voxels. Each voxel has the value of one if it is inside or on the boundary of the chamber. The output is of similar shape and, via thresholding, optionally binary. We further assume that the input is registered to some common anatomical based where the atria is centered via center of mass, and the pulmonary veins are oriented in a consistent manner.

We trained the auto encoder network with 'tied weights' (same weights connecting input and output layers) using Adam [7] on the training set that includes a volume of size 30^3 voxels with 5006 atria. The models were tested on a set of 1384 synthetic atria. Each voxel represents $4[mm^3]$. The sigmoid activation function for all the layers is $\sigma(x) = \frac{1}{1+e^{-x}}$. The network is trained using cross entropy loss [4]; For a training sample z the loss is defined as

$$L(x,z) = \sum_{i=1}^{n} \hat{x}_i \log z_i + (1 - \hat{x}_i) \log(1 - z_i) \tag{1}$$

where summation is over all voxels.

In order to reconstruct a realistic atria volume, we suggest to include *spatial Weights Smoothing Regularization (SWR)*. Our goal is that the weights of the first layer that converts between volumetric input and output (same for the case of tied weights) will be a sufficiently smooth function in R^3 as are heart chambers. We investigated the following loss:

$$L(x,z) + \lambda \sum_{i=1}^{n} \|\nabla_v W_i\|^2 \tag{2}$$

where W denotes the layer weights and the differentiation is with respect to the spatial dimension v. This is defined only in the input and output layers as each weight corresponds to a voxel. The derivative is computed using a finite difference. λ represents how much (if any) regularization is performed.

The problem as defined above can be seen as a segmentation task between the atria interior and exterior regions. In order to assess the performance of the network, we will use the DICE index [8]. In addition, we will examine the resulting boundary, which can be represented as a surface or the set of voxels that separates the interior from exterior. To compare between the generated and the true boundaries, we will use the average of distances between the closest points of the two boundary contours [9] :

$$AVDist(\partial x, \partial y) = 0.5\frac{\sum_{u \in \partial x} \min\{d(u, v) : v \in \partial y\}}{\|\partial x\|} +$$
$$0.5\frac{\sum_{u \in \partial y} \min\{d(u, v) : v \in \partial x\}}{\|\partial y\|} \qquad (3)$$

where $d(a, b)$ is the euclidean distance between voxels a and b.

2.1 Reconstruction Scenarios: Using Sphere Intersection vs An Atria Path

We explore two reconstruction scenarios: in the first, we simulate a case where some volume of space is seen by an imaging modality in a confined region of the atria. The goal is then to complete the full atria based on this region. This could be a clinical setting where the physician visited a specific area with the catheter and would like to an approximation of the whole atria. We create a sphere at a random location. We intersect the sphere with the input left atria and require the network to reconstruct the full input. Figure 2a shows the input red intersected sphere inside the yellow atria. In this scenario we optimize the network architecture for the experiments conducted. Section 3.1 presents the experiment and results of the sphere atria intersection scenario.

In the second scenario, we start with partial data that simulates a catheter path. During a typical electro physiology ablation procedure, the physician maneuvers the catheter from the trans-septal entry point to touch the major pulmonary veins (left and right) for initial anatomy orientation. This maneuver last about a minute. The chosen path for the training was as follows. We begin at the septum which is the entry point during a procedure. The path proceeds to the left superior, left inferior, right inferior and last to right superior PVs. See Fig. 2b for an illustration of the path. We synthesize such path using a graph based algorithm and present the results in Sect. 3.2. In Sect. 3.3 we mimic the path in the lab phantom. Figure 2c shows the two possible generated inputs to the auto-encoder and the desired left atria output.

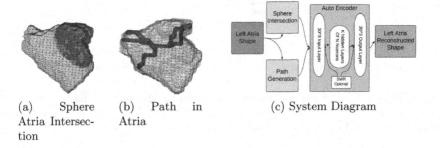

(a)   Sphere Atria Intersection   (b)   Path in Atria   (c) System Diagram

Fig. 2. System and input modalities (Color figure online)

3 Experiments and Results

3.1 Sphere Intersection

We train a network to reconstruct the left atria shape from sphere atria intersection modality (STN). The following training model was used: for each training example a coin was flipped with probability $p = 0.5$. If heads then a ratio $q = 0.5$ of the voxels were set to zero (to preserve auto-encoder properties). Otherwise, a random sphere was created whose center is close enough to the volume center to have a reasonable intersection. Specifically, the center was drawn uniformly from $[0.4 \times 30, 0.7 \times 30]^3$, either with fixed radius $R = 10$ or uniformly $R \in [6, 12]$ and it was intersected with the input volume, setting to zero every voxel outside the sphere. The radius 10 was chosen to cover some part of the atria well but not the other side.

We start with an exploratory phase to select the network architecture based on sphere related experiments, as follows: We conducted a preliminary test to determine a successful choice for the number of neurons in a hidden layer, balancing layer size and performance. We examined networks with a single hidden layer (up to 1000 neurons) that reconstruct from a fixed radius ($R = 10$) sphere intersection. It was found that 500 neurons were optimal. We next trained network architectures with two to four hidden layers with $100, 350, 500$ neurons, with and without the smoothing term, SWR. Training was performed with both fixed and varying intersection radius. Results for reconstruction from different sphere radii intersection are shown for the three best networks with SWR architectures and the best no-SWR architecture, in Fig. 3. Network names are given by the number of neurons per hidden layers - number of hidden layers, S for SWR, NS without and NoVRI stands for fixed radius training. As expected, the overall performance decreases with the sphere radius as the task becomes more challenging. Network 500-3S performs best. Network 350-2NS performance is slightly lower the smooth ones, with increase in the gap as the radius of intersection decreases.

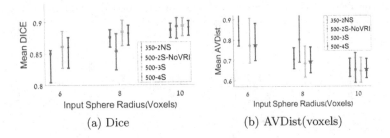

(a) Dice   (b) AVDist(voxels)

Fig. 3. Results for volume completion from different sphere radii intersections. We show the mean as point, and error range for 25% and 75% quantiles. For $R = 6$, 500-2S-NoVRI performance is less than drawing limit.

In Fig. 4 we visualize a median DICE sample for networks 500-3S and 350-2NS. We note that the quality and resemblance to an atria, as well as the shape of the pulmonary veins and ridges, are more evident for the 500-3S, smooth network compared to the bulb generated in network 350-2NS.

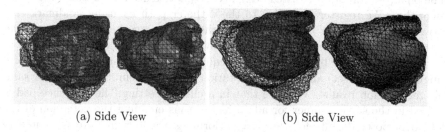

(a) Side View   (b) Side View

Fig. 4. Reconstruction for: (a) 350-2NS and (b) 500-3S, with median DICE score. Red: input volume in ground-truth wire frame; Green: reconstruction result. (Color figure online)

3.2 Synthetic Catheter Path Reconstruction

We next focus on reconstructing the atria shapes using synthetic paths, via path trained networks (PTN). The set of synthesized paths was generated using a novel Dikstra-based algorithm to simulate traversal path between PVs. We provide this description as added material for the interested reader. We start with samples taken along the synthesized paths, and use a set of network configurations, as in the previous section. Table 1 presents the results when starting with the path trained networks, for a variety of architectures, and with/without the spatially-weighted smoothing term (SWR). We compare to the results of the best networks trained using varying sphere intersections (sphere trained network (STN)). Note that for STN with SWR, the path volume was too sparse to activate the network and the result was zero output for most test samples. Thus, they are discarded from the table. From Table 1 we learn that the network 500N-2L is best performing for this task. Including SWR improves the results overall. We see an improvement in results for PTN vs. STN that means that the path information is learned.

Table 1. LA Reconstruction from paths inputs, for PTN compared to STN.

	350N				500N				
	2L		3L		2L		3L		
	SWR	NoSWR	SWR	NoSWR	SWR	NoSWR	SWR	NoSWR	
DICE	0.8494	0.8431	0.8508	0.8008	**0.8521**	0.7589	0.8477	0.8403	Path
AVDist	0.8341	0.83	0.7931	0.9736	**0.7915**	1.129	0.8053	0.8408	Trained
DICE		0.7661		0.7526		0.7449		0.8099	Sphere
AVDist		1.07		1.139		1.167		0.9296	Trained

3.3 Laboratory Phantom

In the final experimental setup, we use an electro-magnetic tracking system to track a catheter tip location in two 3D printed plastic left atria phantoms, recreating paths similar to those described in Sect. 2.1. Figure 5b depicts this scenario. The phantom computer assisted design (CAD) is voxelized using marching cubes algorithm. We register the CAD to the catheter path by using landmark registration. We perform a registration of the coordinates between the tracking system and the anatomical one learned by the network. This registration was performed manually by centering the acquired path and a template path (of a single atria train set) and finding a rotation between them. See Fig. 5c for sample registration results. We note that in a clinical setting, the reference pad is placed in the same manner for all patients - thus enabling the detection of the left atria pose. Results for the best performing architectures are presented in Table 2. Networks are PTN unless stated otherwise. P1 and P2 are phantoms one and two, respectfully, while in parentheses is the number of voxels they occupy. The volume row is the number of voxels the reconstruction had. We can see that 500-3S resulted in adequate reconstruction for P1 while overestimating the volume of P2. However, 500-2S shows a better result for P2 while staggering for P1. Figure 6 depicts the reconstruction results for both phantoms with 500-2S and 500-3S. The locations and orientations of the PVs are detected for all phantoms which is of major clinical importance. The valve direction estimate suffers the most since it is in a region where no path data is available. This induces errors for the networks, impacting DICE and AVDIST performance, as illustrated in the rightmost of each pair of Fig. 6. An additional error source is the difference in PV cut length of the model. Finally, further error is induced due to misalignment in the registration process.

      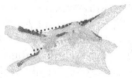

(a) Rigid Phantoms   (b)   CAD   to path   registration   (c)   Phantom   Registration, red is recorded path and blue is template

Fig. 5. Lab system (Color figure online)

Table 2. Rigid phantom results

	500-2S		500-3S		500-3NS		350-2S STN	
	P1(4451)	P2(2194)	P1	P2	P1	P2	P1	P2
DICE	0.7532	**0.7309**	**0.7797**	0.6764	0.7404	0.72	0.6991	0.6636
AVDist	1.4270	**1.328**	**1.2778**	1.6154	1.412	1.3471	1.611	1.4283
Volume	2835	2263	3283	3096	2931	2489	2458	1338

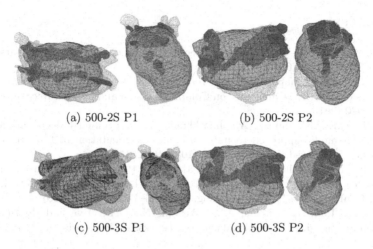

(a) 500-2S P1   (b) 500-2S P2

(c) 500-3S P1   (d) 500-3S P2

Fig. 6. Visualization of reconstruction vs ground truth for 500-3L (top) and 500-2L (bottom) networks, first (a, c) and second (b, d) phantoms. In red is the path. The gray is the ground truth. In cyan is the reconstruction. meshes obtained via marching-cubes. (Color figure online)

4 Conclusions and Future Work

In this work, we demonstrated the capability of an auto-encoder network to learn a complex distinct shape from synthetic dataset. The network is able to recover missing data even for real paths unlike those it was trained for. We view the presented approach as a generalized dictionary based approach where the network actually learns probable atria parts and combines them to recover the missing data. We demonstrated that using spatial weight smoothing regularization (SWR) makes the result of the reconstruction looks more realistic and accurate. Although the reconstruction is not precise as expected, for visualization and the calculation of electrical activation wave it should be adequate, which are the main tasks required by the physician. Promising results were seen in the lab for reconstruction from catheter maneuvers. An actual path performed by a physician contains more information as they usually slide across the boundary to reach the PVs. Therefore, we expect better results once trained on real paths.

We plan to enhance the spatial resolution by combining the network with a CNN. We need to address the issue of rigid transformation to the data from a probable input frame (usual catheter entry locations, known patient poses). We should add a mechanism for refining solution where additional sensor data is available.

References

1. Safran, M., Bar-tal, M.: Model based reconstruction of the heart from sparse samples. US Patent 9,576,107, 21 February 2017
2. Wu, Z., et al.: 3D shapenets: a deep representation for volumetric shapes. In: Proceedings of the IEEE Conference on Computer Vision and Pattern Recognition, pp. 1912–1920 (2015)
3. Avendi, M.R., Kheradvar, A., Jafarkhani, H.: A combined deep-learning and deformable-model approach to fully automatic segmentation of the left ventricle in cardiac MRI. Med. Image Anal. **30**, 108–119 (2016)
4. Vincent, P., Larochelle, H., Bengio, Y., Manzagol, P.-A.: Extracting and composing robust features with denoising autoencoders. In: Proceedings of the 25th International Conference on Machine learning, pp. 1096–1103. ACM (2008)
5. Brock, A., Lim, T., Ritchie, J.M., Weston, N.: Generative and discriminative voxel modeling with convolutional neural networks. arXiv preprint arXiv:1608.04236 (2016)
6. Kingma, D.P., Welling, M.: Auto-encoding variational bayes. Statistics **1050**, 10 (2014)
7. Kingma, D.P., Ba, J.: Adam: a method for stochastic optimization. arXiv preprint arXiv:1412.6980 (2014)
8. Milletari, F., Navab, N., Ahmadi, S.A.: V-net: fully convolutional neural networks for volumetric medical image segmentation. In: 2016 Fourth International Conference on 3D Vision (3DV), pp. 565–571. IEEE (2016)
9. Cha, K.H., Hadjiiski, L., Samala, R.K., Chan, H.-P., Caoili, E.M., Cohan, R.H.: Urinary bladder segmentation in CT urography using deep-learning convolutional neural network and level sets. Med. Phys. **43**(4), 1882–1896 (2016)

High Quality Ultrasonic Multi-line Transmission Through Deep Learning

Sanketh Vedula[1][(✉)], Ortal Senouf[1], Grigoriy Zurakhov[1], Alex Bronstein[1], Michael Zibulevsky[1], Oleg Michailovich[2], Dan Adam[1], and Diana Gaitini[3]

[1] Technion - Israel Institute of Technology, Haifa, Israel
{sanketh,senouf}@campus.technion.ac.il
[2] University of Waterloo, Waterloo, Canada
[3] Rambam Health Care Campus and Faculty of Medicine, Technion, Haifa, Israel

Abstract. Frame rate is a crucial consideration in cardiac ultrasound imaging and 3D sonography. Several methods have been proposed in the medical ultrasound literature aiming at accelerating the image acquisition. In this paper, we consider one such method called *multi-line transmission* (MLT), in which several evenly separated focused beams are transmitted simultaneously. While MLT reduces the acquisition time, it comes at the expense of a heavy loss of contrast due to the interactions between the beams (cross-talk artifact). In this paper, we introduce a data-driven method to reduce the artifacts arising in MLT. To this end, we propose to train an end-to-end convolutional neural network consisting of correction layers followed by a constant apodization layer. The network is trained on pairs of raw data obtained through MLT and the corresponding *single-line transmission* (SLT) data. Experimental evaluation demonstrates significant improvement both in the visual image quality and in objective measures such as contrast ratio and contrast-to-noise ratio, while preserving resolution unlike traditional apodization-based methods. We show that the proposed method is able to generalize well across different patients and anatomies on real and phantom data.

Keywords: Ultrasound imaging · MLT · Deep learning

1 Introduction

Medical ultrasound is a wide-spread imaging modality due to its high temporal resolution, lack of harmful radiation and cost-effectiveness, which distinguishes it from other modalities such as MRI and CT. High frame rate ultrasound is highly desirable for the functional analysis of rapidly moving organs, such as the heart. For a given angular sector size and acquisition depth, the frame rate is limited by the speed of sound in soft tissues (about 1540 m/s). The frame rate depends on the number of transmitted beams needed to cover the field of view; thus, it can be increased by lowering the number of the transmitted events. One such method termed *multi-line acquisition* (MLA) or *parallel receive beamforming* (PRB) employs a smaller number of wide beams in the transmission, and

© Springer Nature Switzerland AG 2018
F. Knoll et al. (Eds.): MLMIR 2018, LNCS 11074, pp. 147–155, 2018.
https://doi.org/10.1007/978-3-030-00129-2_17

constructs a multiple numbers of beams in the reception [14,17]. The drawbacks of the method include block-like artifacts in images, reduced lateral resolution, and reduced contrast [13]. Another high frame-rate method, *multi-line transmission* (MLT), employs a simultaneous transmissions of a multiple number of narrow beams focused in different directions [3,6]. Recently reinvented, this method suffers from a high energy content due to the simultaneous transmissions [15], and from cross-talk artifacts on both the transmit and receive, caused by the interaction between the beams [18,19].

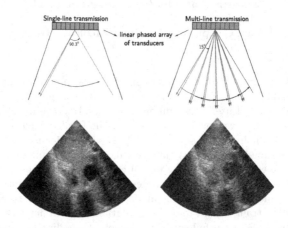

Fig. 1. Single- (left) vs. Multi- (right, with MLT factor of 6) line transmission procedures and their corresponding ultrasound scans. Severe drop in contrast can be observed in the case of MLT. Blue and red lines correspond two consecutive transmissions. (Color figure online)

Over the years, numerous methods were proposed to deal with those artifacts, including constant [18,19] and adaptive [12,22] apodizations, by allocating different frequency bands to different transmissions [1,2], and by using a tissue harmonic mode [11]. The filtered delay-multiply-and-sum beamforming (F-DMAS) [10] was proposed in the context of MLT in [9], demonstrating better artifact rejection, higher contrast ratio (CR) and lateral resolution compared to MLT beamformed with delay-and-sum (DAS) and Tukey apodization on receive, at expense of lower contrast-to-noise ratio (CNR). Finally, short-lag F-DMAS for MLT was studied in [8], demonstrating a contrast improvement for higher maximum-lag values, and resolution and speckle-signal-to-noise ratio (sSNR) improvements for lower lag values, at the expense of decreased MLT cross-talk artifact rejection. By using a simulated 2–MLT, it was demonstrated in [11] that the tissue harmonic imaging mode provides images with a lower transmit cross-talk artifact as compared to the fundamental harmonic imaging. However, the receive cross-talk artifact still requires correction. In the present study, we demonstrate that similarly to the fundamental harmonic, the cross-talk is more severe in the tissue harmonic mode for higher MLT configurations, which is manifested by a lower contrast.

Convolutional neural networks (CNN) were introduced for the processing of ultrasound acquired data in order to generate a high quality plane wave compounding with a reduced number of transmissions [4] as well as for fast despeckling, and CT-quality image generation [20] during the post-processing stage. In a parallel effort, [16] demonstrated the effectiveness of CNNs in improving MLA quality in ultrasound imaging. To the best of our knowledge, ours is the first attempt to use CNN in MLT ultrasound imaging.

Contributions. In this work, we propose an end-to-end CNN-based approach for MLT artifact correction. We train a convolutional neural network consisting of an encoder-decoder architecture followed by a constant apodization layer. The network is trained with dynamically focused element-wise data obtained from *in-vivo* scans in an simulated MLT configuration with the objective to approximate the corresponding single-line transmission (SLT) mode. We demonstrate the performance of our method both qualitatively and quantitatively using metrics such as CR and CNR. Finally, we validate that the trained model generalizes well to different patients, different anatomies, as well as to phantom data.

2   Methods

MLT Simulation. Acquisition of the real MLT data is a complicated task that requires a highly flexible ultrasound system. Fortunately, MLT can be faithfully simulated using the data acquired in a single-line transmit (SLT) mode by summation of the received data prior to the beamforming stage, as was done in [11,12] for the fundamental and tissue harmonic modes. It should be noted that while MLT can be simulated almost perfectly in a fundamental harmonic case, there is a restriction in the tissue harmonic mode due to the nonlinearity of its forward model. It was shown in [11] that in the tissue harmonic mode, the summation of the data sequentially transmitted in two directions provides a good enough approximation for the simultaneous transmission in the same directions if the MLT separation angle is above 15°. The assumption behind the present study is that this approximation holds for a higher MLT number, as long as the separation angle remains the same, since the beam profile between two beams is mainly affected by those beams. For this reason, 4–MLT and 6–MLT with separation angles of 22.6° and 15.06°, respectively, were used in this study.

Clinical use mandates the use of lower excitation voltage in real MLT, implemented in a standard way [15], due to patient safety considerations, which will affect the generation of the tissue harmonic and signal-to-noise ratio (SNR). The latter issue can probably be adressed by the CNNs, that are capable of learning denoising tasks, as has been demonstrated in [21]. It should be noted, that alternative implementations of MLT were proposed in [15], allowing a safer application of the method. However, to the best of our knowledge, no study was performed concerning impact of those methods on image quality. Nevertheless, this study focuses on testing whether the MLT artifact can be corrected using CNN, while the optimization of the number of simultaneous transmissions in the tissue harmonic mode is beyond its scope.

Data Acquisition. For the purpose of the study, we chose imaging of quasi-static internal organs, such as bladder, prostate, and various abdominal structures, since the simulated MLT of the rapidly moving organ may alter the cross-talk artifact. The study was performed with the data acquired using a GE ultra-sound system, scanning 6 healthy human volunteers and a tissue mimicking phantom (GAMMEX Ultrasound 403GS LE Grey Scale Precision Phantom). The tissue harmonic mode was chosen for this study, being a common mode for cardiac imaging, with a contrast resolution that is superior to the fundamental harmonic, at either f_0 or $2f_0$. The scans were performed in a transversal plane by moving a probe in a slow longitudinal motion in order to reduce the correlation in the training data acquired from the same patient. The acquisition frame rate was 18 frames per second. Excitation sinusoidal pulses of 2.56 cycles, centered around $f0 = 1.6$ MHz, were transmitted using a 64-element phased array probe with the pitch of 0.3 mm. No apodization was used on transmit. On receive, the tissue harmonic signal was demodulated (I/Q) at 3.44 MHz and filtered. A 90.3° field-of-view (FOV) was covered with 180 beams. In the case of MLT, the signals were summed element-wise with the appropriate separation angles. Afterward, both SLT and MLT were dynamically focused and summed. In the simulated MLT mode the data were summed after applying a constant apodization window (Tukey, $\alpha = 0.5$) as the best apodization window in [18,19]. At training, non-apodized MLT and SLT data were presented to the network as the input and the desired output, respectively.

Improving MLT Quality Using CNNs. As mentioned earlier, traditional methods tackle the cross-talk artifacts by performing a linear or non-linear processing of a time-delayed element-wise data to reconstruct each pixel in the image. In this work, we propose to replace the traditional pipeline of MLT artifact correction with an end-to-end CNN, as depicted in Fig. 2.

Network Architecture. The proposed network resembles a fully-convolutional autoencoder (albeit different training regime), consisting of 10 layers with symmetric skip connections from each layer in the upsampling track to each layer within the downsampling track [7]. All the convolutions set to 3 × 3, stride 1 and the non-linearities are set to ReLU. Downsampling is performed through average pooling and strided convolutions are used for upsampling. The network accepts time-delayed phase-rotated element-wise I/Q data from the transducer obtained through MLT as the input.

Apodization Stage. A *constant* apodization layer is introduced following the downsampling and upsampling tracks. It is implemented as 1 × 1 convolutions consisting of 64 channels which are applied element-wise and initialized with a boxcar function (window of ones). The layer can be implement any constant apodization such as Tukey or Hann windows.

Training. Following the apodization at the last output stage, the network outputs an artifact-corrected I/Q image. At training, SLT I/Q image are used both to generate a simulated MLT input data as well as the corresponding SLT (artifact-free) reference output. The network is trained as a regressor minimizing the L_1 discrepancy between the predicted network outputs and the corresponding ground-truth SLT data. The loss is minimized using Adam optimizer [5], with the learning rate set to 10^{-4}. The training data were acquired as described in previous sections. A total of 750 frames from the acquired sequences were used for training. The input to the network is a MLT I/Q image of size $696 \times 180 \times 64$ (depth × lines × elements) and the output is an SLT-like I/Q image data of size 696×180 (depth × lines). The training is performed separately for the I and Q components of the image.

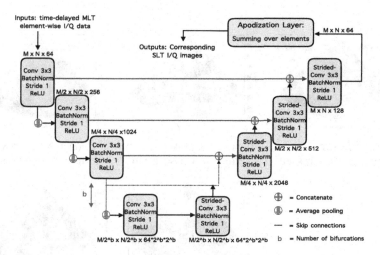

Fig. 2. CNN-based MLT artifact correction pipeline. For all the experiments within this paper: $M = 696, N = 180, b = 5$

3   Experimental Evaluation

Settings. In order to evaluate the performance of the networks trained on 4– and 6–MLT setups, we consider a test set consisting of two frames from the bladder and one frame from a different anatomy acquired from a patient excluded from the training set, and a phantom frame. While all the chosen test frames were unseen during training, the latter two frames portray different image classes that were not part of the training set. The data were acquired as described in Sect. 2. Evaluation was conducted both visually and quantitatively using CR and CNR objective measures as defined in [8].

Results and Discussion. Figure 3 (in the paper) and S1-2 (in the supplementary material)[1] depict the SLT groundtruth, and the artifact-corrected 4– and 6–MLT images. Figure 3 demonstrates a number of anatomical structures in abdominal area, as depicted by the arrows. The CNN processing has restored the CR loss caused by the MLT cross-talk artifact for the 4–MLT, and improved the CR by a 9.8 dB for the 6–MLT, as measured for aorta (yellow contour) and a background region (magenta contour). S1 demonstrates structures in a tissue mimicking phantom, such as anechoic cyst (the black circle marked by a yellow rectangle) and number of a point reflectors. Finally, S2 demonstrates a bladder (large dark cavity) and a prostate, located beneath it, scanned in a transversal plane. The output of our CNN was compared to the MLT image with Tukey ($\alpha = 0.5$) window apodization on receive, a common method to the attenuation of the receive cross-talk artifact.

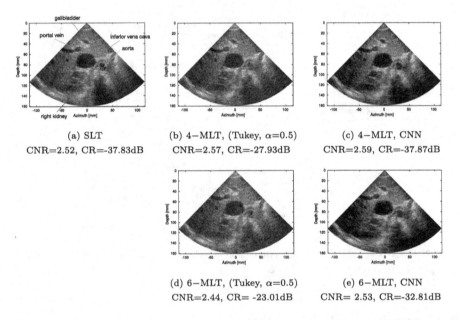

(a) SLT
CNR=2.52, CR=-37.83dB

(b) 4–MLT, (Tukey, α=0.5)
CNR=2.57, CR=-27.93dB

(c) 4–MLT, CNN
CNR=2.59, CR=-37.87dB

(d) 6–MLT, (Tukey, α=0.5)
CNR=2.44, CR= -23.01dB

(e) 6–MLT, CNN
CNR= 2.53, CR=-32.81dB

Fig. 3. CNN-based MLT artifact correction tested on *in-vivo* **abdominal frames** (a) an *in-vivo* frame acquired through SLT from the excluded patient, (b), (d) corresponding 4– and 6–MLT with (Tukey, $\alpha = 0.5$) window, and (c), (e) corresponding CNN-corrected frames

Qualitative evaluation for the phantom frame is presented in S1 along with quantitative measurements, provided in the supplementary materials. A magnified region depicts the response from one of the wires of the phantom. A thinner appearance, as compared to the apodized MLT image, can be observed for both

---

[1] The supplementary materual can be found here https://drive.google.com/open?id=1fNq_NHG_ye1Ph6Yvuxvr-y8a_L3cXofE.

4– and 6–MLT frames processed with the proposed CNN, since no apodization was needed to attenuate the artifacts. Quantitatively, the CR of the anechoic cyst as compared to the nearby tissue, was restored for the case of 6–MLT, whereas for the 4–MLT case it was improved by almost 7 dB as compared to the SLT. Since the network was trained on the data with a higher number of a strong reflectors, thus higher artifact content, it is possible that the artifact content is overestimated in some cases. The images of the bladder (S2) appear to have a higher quality in the 4–MLT and 6–MLT CNN corrected cases, as compared to the respective apodized versions. Quantitatively, the improvement in contrast over apodized MLT was around 10 dB for 4-MLT and 13 dB for 6–MLT.

A slight CNR improvement as compared to the apodized MLT was measured in all cases, except for the 6–MLT for the tissue mimicking phantom, where the CNR remained the same. The performance of our CNN, verified on the testing set frames of internal organs, and of a tissue mimicking phantom, suggests that it generalizes well to other scenes and patients, despite being trained on a small dataset of bladder frames.

It should be noted that the coherent processing of the data (through convolutions applied on the data prior to the envelope detection) along the lateral direction may impose motion artifacts while imaging regions involving rapid movement (such as cardiac tissue and blood). Nevertheless, in most compensation methods, the correction is performed without relying on the adjacent samples in lateral direction, thus, similar approaches relying on constraints in the lateral direction can be built into the neural network. We defer this case to a future studies.

4 Conclusion

In this paper, we have demonstrated that correction provided by an end-to-end CNN outperforms the constant apodization-based correction method of MLT cross-talk artifacts, as measured using CR and CNR. Moreover, the obtained CNN generalizes well for different anatomical scenes. In the future, we intend to address the problem of MLT artifact suppression for rapidly moving objects scenes, by training a CNN to correct all the lines beamformed from a single transmit event. Furthermore, we aim at exploring the possibility of similarly reconstructing artifact-free images for combined MLT-MLA configurations, that introduce an even larger boost in frame rate.

Acknowledgments. This research was partially supported by ERC StG RAPID.

References

1. Demi, L., Ramalli, A., Giannini, G., Mischi, M.: In vitro and in vivo tissue harmonic images obtained with parallel transmit beamforming by means of orthogonal frequency division multiplexing. IEEE Trans. Ultrason. Ferroelectr. Freq. Control **62**(1), 230–235 (2015)

2. Demi, L., Verweij, M., Van Dongen, K.W.: Parallel transmit beamforming using orthogonal frequency division multiplexing applied to harmonic imaging-a feasibility study. IEEE Trans. Ultrason. Ferroelectr. Freq. Control (2012)
3. Drukarev, A., Konstantinides, K., Seroussi, G.: Beam transformation techniques for ultrasonic medical imaging. IEEE Trans. Ultrason. Ferroelectr. Freq. Control 40(6), 717–726 (1993)
4. Gasse, M., Millioz, F., Roux, E., Garcia, D., Liebgott, H., Friboulet, D.: High-quality plane wave compounding using convolutional neural networks. IEEE Trans. Ultrason. Ferroelectr. Freq. Control 64(10), 1637–1639 (2017)
5. Kingma, D.P., Ba, J.: Adam: a method for stochastic optimization. In: ICLR (2015)
6. Mallart, R., Fink, M.: Improved imaging rate through simultaneous transmission of several ultrasound beams. In: New Developments in Ultrasonic Transducers and Transducer Systems. International Society for Optics and Photonics (1992)
7. Mao, X., Shen, C., Yang, Y.: Image restoration using very deep convolutional encoder-decoder networks with symmetric skip connections. In: NIPS (2016)
8. Matrone, G., Ramalli, A.: Spatial coherence of backscattered signals in multi-line transmit ultrasound imaging and its effect on short-lag filtered-delay multiply and sum beamforming. Appl. Sci. 8(4), 486 (2018)
9. Matrone, G., Ramalli, A., Savoia, A.S., Tortoli, P., Magenes, G.: High frame-rate, high resolution ultrasound imaging with multi-line transmission and filtered-delay multiply and sum beamforming. IEEE Trans. Med. Imaging (2017)
10. Matrone, G., Savoia, A.S., Caliano, G., Magenes, G.: The delay multiply and sum beamforming algorithm in ultrasound B-mode medical imaging. IEEE Trans. Med. Imaging 34(4), 940–949 (2015)
11. Prieur, F., Denarie, B., Austeng, A., Torp, H.: Correspondence-multi-line transmission in medical imaging using the second-harmonic signal. IEEE Trans. Ultrason. Ferroelectr. Freq. Control 60(12), 2682–2692 (2013)
12. Rabinovich, A., Feuer, A., Friedman, Z.: Multi-line transmission combined with minimum variance beamforming in medical ultrasound imaging. IEEE Trans. Ultrason. Ferroelectr. Freq. Control 62(5), 814–827 (2015)
13. Rabinovich, A., Friedman, Z., Feuer, A.: Multi-line acquisition with minimum variance beamforming in medical ultrasound imaging. IEEE Trans. Ultrason. Ferroelectr. Freq. Control 60(12), 2521–2531 (2013)
14. Ramm, O.T.V., Smith, S.W., Pavy, H.G.: High-speed ultrasound volumetric imaging system. II. parallel processing and image display. IEEE Trans. Ultrason. Ferroelectr. Freq. Control 38(2), 109–115 (1991)
15. Santos, P., Tong, L., Ortega, A., Løvstakken, L., Samset, E., Dhooge, J.: Acoustic output of multi-line transmit beamforming for fast cardiac imaging: a simulation study. IEEE Trans. Ultrason. Ferroelectr. Freq. Control (2015)
16. Senouf, O., et al.: High frame-rate cardiac ultrasound imaging with deep learning. In: MICCAI (2018)
17. Shattuck, D.P., Weinshenker, M.D., Smith, S.W., von Ramm, O.T.: Explososcan: a parallel processing technique for high speed ultrasound imaging with linear phased arrays. Acous. Soc. Am. J. 75, 1273–1282 (1984)
18. Tong, L., Gao, H., D'hooge, J.: Multi-transmit beam forming for fast cardiac imaging-a simulation study. IEEE Trans. Ultrason. Ferroelectr. Freq. Control 60(8), 1719–1731 (2013)
19. Tong, L., Ramalli, A., Jasaityte, R., Tortoli, P., D'hooge, J.: Multi-transmit beam forming for fast cardiac imagingexperimental validation and in vivo application. IEEE Trans. Med. Imaging 33(6), 1205–1219 (2014)

20. Vedula, S., Senouf, O., Bronstein, A., Michailovich, O., Zibulevsky, M.: Towards CT-quality Ultrasound Imaging using Deep Learning. arXiv preprint arXiv:1710.06304 (2017)
21. Zhang, K., Zuo, W., Chen, Y., Meng, D., Zhang, L.: Beyond a Gaussian denoiser: residual learning of deep CNN for image denoising. IEEE Trans. Image Process. **26**(7), 3142–3155 (2017)
22. Zurakhov, G., Tong, L., Ramalli, A., Tortoli, P., Dhooge, J., Friedman, Z., Adam, D.: Multi line transmit beamforming combined with adaptive apodization. IEEE Trans. Ultrason. Ferroelectr. Freq. Control (2018)

Author Index

Printed in the United States
By Bookmasters